ADOLESCENT MEDICINE: STATE OF THE ART REVIEWS

Evaluation & Management of Adolescent Issues

GUEST EDITOR

Alain Joffe, MD, MPH

April 2008 • Volume 19 • Number 1

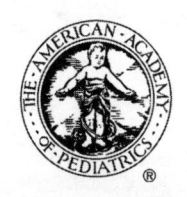

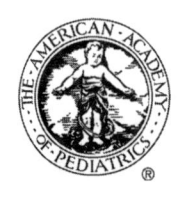

ADOLESCENT MEDICINE CLINICS:
STATE OF THE ART REVIEWS
April 2008
Editor: Diane E. Beausoleil
Marketing Manager: Linda Smessaert
Production Manager: Shannan Martin

Volume 19, Number 1
ISBN 978-1-58110-288-8
ISSN 1934-4287
MA0434
SUB1006

Copyright © 2008 American Academy of Pediatrics. All rights reserved. No part of this publication may be reproduced or transmitted in any form or by any means, electronic or mechanical, including photocopying, recording, or any information retrieval system, without written permission from the Publisher (fax the permissions editor at 847/434-8780).

Adolescent Medicine: State of the Art Reviews is published three times per year by the American Academy of Pediatrics, 141 Northwest Point Blvd, Elk Grove Village, IL 60007-1098. Periodicals postage paid at Arlington Heights, IL.

POSTMASTER: Send address changes to American Academy of Pediatrics, Department of Marketing and Publications, Attn: AM:STARs, 141 Northwest Point Blvd, Elk Grove Village, IL 60007-1098.

Subscriptions: Subscriptions to *Adolescent Medicine: State of the Art Reviews* (AM:STARs) are provided to members of the American Academy of Pediatrics' Section on Adolescent Health as part of annual section membership dues. All others, please contact the AAP Customer Service Center at 866/843-2271 (7:00 am–5:30 pm Central Time, Monday–Friday) for pricing and information.

Adolescent Medicine: State of the Art Reviews

Official Journal of the American Academy of Pediatrics
Section on Adolescent Health

EDITORS-IN-CHIEF

Victor C. Strasburger, MD
Professor of Pediatrics
Chief, Division of Adolescent
Medicine
University of New Mexico
School of Medicine
Albuquerque, New Mexico

Donald E. Greydanus, MD
Professor of Pediatrics
Michigan State University and
Pediatrics Program Director
Kalamazoo Center for Medical
Studies
Kalamazoo, Michigan

ASSOCIATE EDITORS

Robert T. Brown, MD
Columbus, Ohio

Paula K. Braverman, MD
Cincinnati, Ohio

Susan M. Coupey, MD
Bronx, New York

Manuel Schydlower, MD
El Paso, Texas

Martin M. Fisher, MD
Manhasset, New York

Alain Joffe, MD, MPH
Baltimore, Maryland

EVALUATION & MANAGEMENT OF ADOLESCENT ISSUES

EDITORS-IN-CHIEF

VICTOR C. STRASBURGER, MD, Professor of Pediatrics, Division of Adolescent Medicine, University of New Mexico, School of Medicine, Albuquerque, New Mexico

DONALD E. GREYDANUS, MD, Professor of Pediatrics, Michigan State University; and Pediatrics Program Director, Kalamazoo Center for Medical Studies, Kalamazoo, Michigan

GUEST EDITOR

ALAIN JOFFE, MD, MPH, Student Health and Wellness Center, Johns Hopkins University, Baltimore, Maryland

CONTRIBUTORS

MARVIN E. BELZER, MD, Division of Adolescent Medicine, Childrens Hospital Los Angeles, Los Angeles, California

CAROL J. BLAISDELL, MD, Department of Pediatrics and Physiology, University of Maryland School of Medicine, Baltimore, Maryland

KRISTIN DELISI, CRNP, Division of Adolescent Medicine, Children's Hospital of Pittsburgh, University of Pittsburgh Medical Center, Pittsburgh, Pennsylvania

KATE FOTHERGILL, PhD, Department of Health, Behavior, and Society, Johns Hopkins Bloomberg School of Public Health, Baltimore, Maryland

MELANIE A. GOLD, DO, Division of Adolescent Medicine, Department of Pediatrics, University of Pittsburgh School of Medicine, Pittsburgh, Pennsylvania

RENEE FLAX-GOLDENBERG, MD, Division of Pediatric Radiology, Department of Radiology, Johns Hopkins Medical Institutions, Baltimore, Maryland

DEBRA K. KATZMAN, MD, FRCP(C), Division of Adolescent Medicine, Department of Pediatrics, Hospital for Sick Children and University of Toronto, Toronto, Ontario, Canada

JOHN R. KNIGHT, Division on Addictions and Department of Pediatrics, Harvard Medical School; Center for Adolescent Substance Abuse Research, Division of Developmental Medicine, Division of Adolescent/Young Adult Medicine, and Department of Psychiatry, Children's Hospital Boston, Boston, Massachusetts

PATRICIA K. KOKOTAILO, MD, MPH, Department of Pediatrics, University of Wisconsin School of Medicine and Public Health, Madison, Wisconsin

RICHARD E. KREIPE, MD, Division of Adolescent Medicine, Department of Pediatrics, Golisano Children's Hospital at Strong, University of Rochester, Rochester, New York

SHARON LEVY, MD, MPH, Department of Pediatrics, Harvard Medical School; Center for Adolescent Substance Abuse Research, Division of Developmental Medicine, and Department of Psychiatry, Children's Hospital Boston, Boston, Massachusetts

CHRISTIAN D. NAGY, MD, Division of Pediatric Cardiology, Department of Pediatrics, The Helen B. Taussig Congenital Heart Disease Center, Johns Hopkins University School of Medicine, Baltimore, Maryland

CHRISTOPHER M. OBERHOLZER, MD, Department of Pediatrics, Division of Pediatric Infectious Diseases, University of Rochester School of Medicine and Dentistry, Rochester, New York

JOHANNA OLSON, MD, Division of Adolescent Medicine, Childrens Hospital Los Angeles, Los Angeles, California

RHEANNA PLATT, MD, MPH, Department of Pediatrics, Johns Hopkins School of Medicine, Baltimore, Maryland

OLLE JANE Z. SAHLER, MD, Departments of Pediatrics, Psychiatry, Medical Humanities, and Oncology, University of Rochester School of Medicine and Dentistry, and Division of Pediatric Hematology/Oncology, Golisano Children's Hospital at Strong, Rochester, New York

LAUREN SPIKER, MEd, Melissa's Living Legacy Teen Cancer Foundation, Rochester, New York

CATHLEEN STEINEGGER, MD, Department of Pediatrics, Hospital for Sick Children and University of Toronto, Toronto, Ontario, Canada

W. REID THOMPSON, MD, Division of Pediatric Cardiology, Department of Pediatrics, The Helen B. Taussig Congenital Heart Disease Center, Johns Hopkins University School of Medicine, Baltimore, Maryland

MELANIE WELLINGTON, MD, PhD, Department of Pediatrics, Division of Pediatric Infectious Diseases, University of Rochester School of Medicine and Dentistry, Rochester, New York

LAWRENCE S. WISSOW, MD, MPH, Berman Bioethics Institute, Johns Hopkins University, Baltimore, Maryland

EVALUATION & MANAGEMENT OF ADOLESCENT ISSUES

CONTENTS

Preface   xiii
Alain Joffe

Introduction to Interviewing: The Art of Communicating With Adolescents   1
Richard E. Kreipe

> Detailed descriptions of a variety of skills, techniques, and tools that facilitate communication with an adolescent in health care settings are the focus of this article. An understanding of developmental tasks of adolescence developmental tasks include pubertal status, autonomy (control, confidentiality, and adherence), identity, and cognitive features (egocentrism, personal fable, and imaginary audience). Common pitfalls in interviewing adolescents are described along with ways to avoid them. Consideration of the nature and setting of the visit also helps to frame the interview. Effective communication with adolescents helps to build a therapeutic alliance and makes interactions more rewarding. Skills that underlie effective communication with adolescents include applying principles of adolescent development; self-awareness; a nonjudgmental approach; flexibility with consistency; active listening; and observing. Techniques that enhance an adolescent's information-sharing include engaging patients as therapeutic allies; initiating the interview with nonthreatening topics; assuming nothing; clarifying any inferences made; providing confidentiality and including the patient in the collection of data from other sources; confronting passive-aggressive behavior and substituting assertiveness; asking the patient to keep a daily journal; providing patients with options from which to choose when discussing abstract concepts; linking potentially embarrassing questions with health; using reflective responses; using summarizing statements; and making use of body language.

Interviewing the Adolescent With an Eating Disorder   18
Cathleen Steinegger, Debra K. Katzman

> The initial encounter with an adolescent with an eating disorder and his or her family represents an opportunity to begin to understand the patient's problem, establish a therapeutic relationship,

and determine a diagnosis. In this article we provide the basic principles of interviewing an adolescent with an eating disorder: how to approach the interview, how to engage the patient, the types of questions to ask, how to ask these questions, and, finally, how to pull the information together to establish a diagnosis and treatment plan. We use examples throughout the article to highlight the unique nature and complexities of interviewing an adolescent with an eating disorder. A successful interview can be a rewarding experience. Interviewing the adolescent with an eating disorder is the first step toward recovery.

Talking With Adolescents and Their Families About Emotional and Behavioral Concerns 41
Rheanna Platt, Kate Fothergill, Lawrence S. Wissow

Up to one quarter of US adolescents are thought to have mental health problems, a proportion that seems to be increasing. Only a minority of these adolescents reportedly receive treatment, but of those who do, for many it is in the context of primary care. This article addresses 4 challenges commonly encountered by primary care providers who treat adolescents: (1) working with/responding to adolescents' potentially limited or biased knowledge of mental health problems and their treatment; (2) balancing adolescents' desire for confidentiality with families' interests in being involved in the adolescents' care; (3) managing encounters with families and adolescents together, especially when the adolescent is a reluctant participant; and (4) working with families who are discouraged or feel hopeless.

Motivational Interviewing With Adolescents 54
Patricia K. Kokotailo, Melanie A. Gold

Adolescents often engage in health behaviors that can pose a threat to their health. Traditional approaches to encouraging adolescents to change these behaviors, such as providing information about possible risks or simply advising them to stop, are ineffective at best and counterproductive at worst. In this article we describe an alternative approach, motivational interviewing, that enhances the adolescent's own intrinsic capacity for change by creating or identifying discrepancies between the adolescent's personal goals and behaviors that could interfere with achieving those goals. We review the fundamental principles of motivational interviewing, describe basic strategies and techniques that clinicians can use in working with adolescents, and review the evidence supporting its use in this age group.

Motivational Interviewing and Sexual and Contraceptive Behaviors 69
Melanie A. Gold, Kristin Delisi

> Unintended pregnancy and sexually transmitted diseases are among the greatest health care problems facing young men and women in the United States. Health care providers are in a unique position to address young people's risk of unintended pregnancy and sexually transmitted diseases, yet evidence for effective counseling strategies is limited. Motivational interviewing is a theory-based behavior-counseling style that provides a promising approach to addressing many risk-taking behaviors in youths. Application of motivational interviewing to sexual and contraceptive counseling can be used to identify discrepancies between goals or values and current behaviors and can support young people's decision-making and confidence in using contraceptive methods. In this article, we use a case-based approach to demonstrate how motivational interviewing can be applied to the following situations: an adolescent girl who is ambivalent about initiating sexual activity; an adolescent boy who uses condoms inconsistently; an adolescent who is ambivalent about becoming pregnant; and an adolescent who is uncertain about initiating hormonal contraception.

Helping Adolescents to Stop Using Drugs: Role of the Primary Care Clinician 83
Sharon Levy, John R. Knight

> Substance use in common during adolescence. Health maintenance visits provide an ideal opportunity to screen, assess, treat and/or refer teenagers to reduce alcohol and drug use and related consequences. This article uses case vignettes to demonstrate effective strategies to assess and treat substance use by adolescents using very brief interventions based on motivational interviewing, which are practical for use during health maintenance appointments.

Adherence in Adolescents: A Review of the Literature 99
Marvin E. Belzer, Johanna Olson

> Adherence to medication is a complex phenomena that has a major impact on health outcomes. Medication adherence in adolescents has a wide but incomplete body of literature that is frequently linked to chronic illnesses. This chapter reviews the adolescent adherence literature and adresses how to measure adherence, factors associated with adherence and nonadherence, interventions to improve adherence and research findings

on adherence in selected chronic conditions such as human immunodeficiency virus (HIV) infection, organ transplant, asthma, contraception and diabetes mellitus.

Communicating With Teens Who Are Living With Cancer   119
Olle Jane Z. Sahler, Lauren Spiker

Communicating with adolescents who have life-threatening illness includes not only providing them with information about their condition but also involving them in management from the moment of diagnosis to the moment of death if their illness is terminal. In this article, cancer provides the context for the story of one young woman as told by her mother. Although the specific experiences recounted are highly personal, they illustrate many of the principles of communication important to the provision of good care and caring during extraordinarily difficult times: When and how much should the teen patient be told and by whom? How much should the teen participate in decision-making and about which issues? What are dying teens most concerned about and how should physicians respond to their questions, fears, and hopes? And, very importantly, what motivates a person to become a physician and how does his/her humanness influence thoughts, feelings, and behaviors when confronting the need to not only deliver, but also personally cope with, bad news?

Serological Diagnosis of Infectious Diseases in the Adolescent   135
Christopher M. Oberholzer, Melanie Wellington

As adolescents begin to gain their independence, they engage in behaviors that can result in exposure to infectious diseases such as Epstein-Barr virus, cytomegalovirus, hepatitis, HIV, syphilis, and Lyme disease. Serology is the mainstay of diagnosis for many of these infections. Serological assays may also be useful screening tools for detecting asymptomatic disease in adolescents at high risk. The majority of serological assays are based on detecting host antibody responses to infection. An understanding of the natural history of this process is useful for the clinician, because it facilitates detection of exposure, ongoing infection, and/or immunity to pathogens. In this article we discuss the common serological tests and their interpretation for important infectious conditions that are frequently encountered by adolescent patients.

Pulmonary Function Testing in the Adolescent 149
Carol J. Blaisdell

Pulmonary function testing can be used as an objective measure of lung function in adolescents and young adults with known or suspected lung disease. The choice of an appropriate objective and reproducible test of lung function can often confirm a working diagnosis in the clinician's evaluation. In addition, lung function testing is important for assessing progression of lung disease and response to therapy. This article reviews the principles and interpretation of lung function testing in adolescents, including peak expiratory flow rates, spirometry, lung volumes, response to bronchodilators, and testing to confirm airway hyperresponsiveness.

Cardiac Testing in Adolescents 169
Christian D. Nagy, W. Reid Thompson

Diagnostic testing in adolescents and young adults with known or suspected heart disease typically involves the use of electrocardiography, various imaging modalities such as echocardiography, and laboratory investigations. Authors discuss common tests that may be requested by the generalist or cardiologist to evaluate the heart. The emphasis is on indications for ordering a specific test, understanding their strengths and weaknesses, and basic interpretation of the results. Heart disease in adolescents primarily includes previously diagnosed congenital lesions, undiagnosed defects such as atrial septal defect (ASD) or aortic valve abnormalities that are often asymptomatic in childhood, inherited latent conditions that may first become mainfest during the teen years, such as hypertrophic cardiomyopathy (HCM), and acquired disease such as myocarditis. Signs and symptoms of possible heart disease, when present, may include a pathological murmur or heart sound(s), chest pain and shortness of breath, especially when associated with exercise, other signs of heart failure, palpitations or syncope. An electrocardiogram is often ordered by the generalist or specialist to evaluate symptoms of possible heart disease. Most imaging studies, including echocardiography, are ordered or performed by the cardiologist to diagnose specific defects conditions, and catheterizations are increasingly done primarily for intervention purposes.

Imaging in Adolescent Medicine 193

Renee Flax-Goldenberg

Choosing the best imaging study for some of the common clinical entities encountered in the adolescent population is challenging. In all cases, a thorough history and physical examination are the foundation for arriving at a concise differential diagnosis. The purpose of imaging should be to confirm or rule out suspected pathology that requires immediate intervention or to further narrow the differential and direct additional imaging investigation accordingly. The topics for this article include suspected appendicitis, severe headache, acute-onset chest pain, acute-onset scrotal pain, lower abdominal and pelvic pain in adolescent girls, and suspected nephrolithiasis.

Index 203

Preface

Evaluation & Management of Adolescent Issues

Practitioners of adolescent medicine know all too well that evaluating an adolescent's presenting symptom and identifying the underlying basis for it can often prove challenging, requiring a sensitive and thoughtful diagnostic interview and judicious use of diagnostic tests. Even when the chief concern becomes apparent or the diagnosis clear, engaging youth and their families in a therapeutic plan is not always straightforward. These challenges – while at times frustrating – are one of the attractions of adolescent medicine.

This issue focuses on these aspects of clinical care. Just as we have learned more about the various disease entities that occur during adolescence, so, too, have we learned more about how to communicate with, evaluate, and manage effectively adolescents in our care. Each chapter is written by experts who draw upon the latest information in the field. The first eight chapters focus on critical aspects of communicating with adolescents and their families and partnering with them to achieve therapeutic goals. The first chapter provides an overview of communicating with adolescents, followed by several chapters addressing specific aspects of interviewing or engaging adolescents with some of the most challenging illnesses adolescent medicine specialists are likely to face: the adolescent with a suspected eating disorder, the adolescent who is using drugs, and the adolescent who is living with cancer. This last chapter is unique in that it is co-authored by a pediatric hematologist-oncologist and the mother of a teenager who died from cancer. An additional chapter focuses on working with teenagers (and their families) whose primary problems are emotional and/or behavioral concerns; another provides an overview of adherence to medical regimens, with specific emphasis on improving adherence among adolescents.

Motivational interviewing, an approach to effecting behavior change, has been shown to be very effective with adults. Emerging research, as outlined in two chapters in this issue, suggests this approach may be equally effective with adolescents. Chapter four provides an overview of the principles of motivational interviewing while chapter five demonstrates how these principles can be applied to counseling teenagers about sexual behaviors.

No matter how skillful a clinician may be at communicating with adolescents, there are times when he/she will require use of diagnostic testing to confirm a

Copyright © 2008 American Academy of Pediatrics. All rights reserved. ISSN 1934-4287

diagnosis or manage a patient. The last four chapters cover approaches to diagnostic testing that adolescent medicine clinicians are likely to utilize in daily practice: serologic testing for suspected infections, pulmonary function testing, cardiac testing, and diagnostic imaging. The authors review the latest information on a wide variety of diagnostic tests specific to symptoms or illnesses that are likely to present during adolescence.

I learned a great deal from reading all of these chapters. I hope that you, too, will find them useful in your clinical work with adolescents.

Alain Joffe, MD, MPH
Student Health and Wellness Center
Johns Hopkins University
Baltimore, Maryland

Introduction to Interviewing: The Art of Communicating With Adolescents

Richard E. Kreipe, MD*

Division of Adolescent Medicine, Department of Pediatrics, Golisano Children's Hospital at Strong, University of Rochester, 601 Elmwood Avenue, Box 690, Rochester, NY 14642, USA

This article addresses skills and techniques for facilitating communication with an adolescent in health care settings. Following a practical description of 3 developmental tasks of adolescence related to interviewing, there follows a detailed exploration of key concepts related to effective communication with adolescents that focus on tools, skills, and techniques, as well as common pitfalls. Consideration of the nature and setting of the visit help to frame the interview. Effective communication with adolescents helps to build a therapeutic alliance and makes interactions more rewarding. When the terms "physician" or "medical" are used in this article, the concepts are applicable to other health care professionals in a variety of settings.

DEVELOPMENTAL TASKS OF ADOLESCENTS RELEVANT TO INTERVIEWING ADOLESCENTS

Pubertal Status

Physical maturation of puberty does not always correlate with cognitive or emotional maturity. Early-developing adolescents grow more rapidly and may appear chronologically older than their later-developing peers. Similarly, those with a chronic illness may have delayed pubertal maturation and appear younger. If a patient looks much younger or older than his or her chronologic age, one might say, "I know that you are 14 years old, but I wonder if people sometimes treat you like you are 12 (or 16), because you may look younger (or older) than you are?" A positive response can be followed with, "What's good, or bad, about that?"

Adolescents may feel awkward and self-conscious, especially when pubertal changes occur rapidly. Informing the patient in advance of what will and will not occur during

---

*Corresponding author.
E-mail address: richard_kreipe@urmc.rochester.edu (R. E. Kreipe).

Copyright © 2008 American Academy of Pediatrics. All rights reserved. ISSN 1934-4287

the encounter can mitigate worries. Routine annual physical examinations have a low yield in detecting new pathology and low cost-effectiveness.[1,2] However, if there is a pertinent history (eg, sexual activity) or symptoms (eg, knee pain), then an examination is indicated. If a patient is apprehensive about an examination, engaging them in an interview during the physical examination can facilitate the interview process, as described below. Combining physical examination with interview is especially useful for situations in which the practitioner is on a tight time schedule and allows key elements of the history-taking and physical examination to be performed at the same time.

To start the physical examination, one can palpate the adolescent's head while inquiring about helmet use: "Do you ride a bike, skateboard, or ATV [all-terrain vehicle]? Do you always wear safety equipment?" If the adolescent does keep physically active and wear safety equipment, one can provide positive feedback: "Good for you! Some of my patients don't like to wear them, but it's a good idea to wear a helmet anytime you get on a bike." When examining the lungs, one can ask about tobacco exposure, including secondhand smoke: "Before I listen to your lungs, do you have any problems breathing? Some of my patients your age smoke or are around others who smoke. Do you or your parents smoke? What about your friends?"

In the course of the musculoskeletal examination, one could comment, "As I examine your muscles and joints, I wonder what kind of physical activity you like to do? Do you play sports? On organized teams or just with friends? Do you have any regular exercise routine? What's it like?" One should not ask only about "popular" sports or assume that adolescents with physical disabilities do not engage in sports. Adolescents with special health care needs might be limited in their activities more by their parents than their abilities. Focus on abilities more than limitations.

When examining the skin, one can note a number of things: "Do you ever go tanning? How often?" or "You have fair skin. Do you ever use sun blockers when you are outside?" or "I see that you have a tattoo here, do you have any others?"[3] or "When did you get your nose pierced? Any other places that you have had pierced? Any problems with any of the piercings?" A nonjudgmental approach to positive responses will keep the lines of communication open.

Autonomy

The index of Steinberg's classic textbook *Adolescence*[4] has an entire chapter devoted to "autonomy" but none devoted to "independence." Gilligan[5] and others have demonstrated that for many adolescents, especially girls, the construct of independence is associated with feeling isolated, alone, or abandoned. Therefore, many adults function at a higher level when they recognize that they are part of a network of interdependent, but autonomous, relationships.

Control

Because perception of autonomy may be linked to a sense of being in control, it is useful to begin a visit when the patient is referred for consultation by explicitly noting respect for autonomy. When first meeting a patient, especially if he or she appears unhappy about being in a consultation clinic, one can start by introducing one's self and determining what name the patient wants to be called. The next statement might be, "Some patients are here because they want to work on a health issue, some are only here because their parents make them come, and for some it's a little bit of each. I'm interested in the part of you that wants to be here, as well as the part that doesn't. Let's start by talking about the part that doesn't want to be here first, because that part will interfere with our working together. Then we can talk about the part that wants to be here, especially about what you would like to get out of today's visit."

This opening gambit resulted in a response from Cheryl, a 15-year-old girl with type 1 diabetes: "I'm only here because my mother dragged me here. This is so stupid. She's the one with the problem." Cheryl's goal for the visit was to "get my mother off my back." Her mother's response was, "I want you to get her to take better control of her diabetes," or "She doesn't listen to me about anything, I hope you can get through to her." When control struggles are prominent, label them appropriately: "I know that her school nurse wanted me to see Cheryl because she's worried about her sugar control, but my sense is that you are both frustrated about fighting with each other about her diabetes all the time. Does fighting seem to make things better or worse?" With consensus that fighting only makes things worse, a mutually agreeable and reasonable goal might be to have Cheryl work with the physician to gradually lower her hemoglobin A_{1C} levels while the mother backs off from her authoritarian stance to take a more supportive one.

Control issues can also relate to excessive compliance or open resistance: "Some of my patients tell me what they think is the right answer or what I want to hear. Sometimes they are embarrassed about things that they do. The only thing I ask of my patients is to be honest and tell me things as they see them." Adolescents who are not interested in being part of the interview (resisters) may answer questions with "I don't know." It is useful to say, "I've noticed that you answer a lot of my questions with 'I don't know.' This can mean different things: 'I don't understand the question'—which is my problem for not making myself understood—or 'I don't want to talk about it' or 'I don't know the answer to your question.' If you don't understand the question, please tell me that. If you don't want to talk about it, let me know that, too. That way, we both can agree that 'I don't know' means 'I don't know.' Okay?"

Confidentiality

The importance of confidentiality cannot be overestimated in conducting the interview and should be discussed at the outset of a new relationship with an adolescent patient. Klein et al[6] found that adolescents whose providers did not discuss confidentiality were more likely to report having withheld information about their health behaviors than those whose providers discussed confidentiality. The findings agree with that of a strong link between the perception of confidentiality in health care and the decision of teens to seek health care.[7] Likewise, Lehrer et al[8] recently reported that adolescents who engage in health risk behaviors, compared with those who do not, are more likely to avoid health care because of concerns about confidentiality. Finally, Ford et al[9] found that adolescents know far less about the protections of confidentiality than about the limits.

Thus, comments about the limitations of confidentiality need to be balanced with reassurance about the protection of confidentiality: "What we talk about will be kept private unless I believe that you might harm yourself or others. Then, we would need to work together to figure out who else needs to be included for me to help you best." With respect to protection of confidentiality: "Some patients are afraid to talk to a doctor about sex or drugs because they think that whatever they say will get back to their parents. Those are things that can be kept private. As I said before, I won't go behind your back, but I will let you know when I think your health or safety is in danger because of information that you want kept confidential."

When adolescents "don't want their parents to know," it is often related to embarrassment about disclosing the details of their behavior. For example, an adolescent with bulimia nervosa may be reluctant to disclose self-induced vomiting after secretive binge eating and self-injurious behaviors related to mood disturbance. A physician in a health service could respond, "Suzanne, you've said that you don't want your parents to know anything about your eating disorder and that you're only here because your sorority sisters threatened to tell your parents if you didn't come to see me. But, I'm concerned about your binge eating and vomiting and cutting, and I believe that there's at least a small part of you that wants help. We don't have to specifically talk about behaviors with your parents at first. We can focus on general issues, like how you don't feel very good about your body and are depressed, and I'll be there to help."

Adherence

A normalizing statement may facilitate talking about treatment adherence: "It can be hard to remember to take medicines (go to therapy, etc) regularly. It may interfere with things you would like to do or make you feel different, adults nag you about it, or you just forget. Are any of those reasons true for you? How often do you miss taking your medications (or treatment, etc)? Are there things that you think you (or others) could do to make it easier to follow through with what has been recommended?" This helps to establish a therapeutic alliance, with the physician and patient sharing common goals.

Identity

Acknowledging the importance of peer-group influences can help to frame health education messages embedded in the interview: "You say that some of your friends smoke but that you don't yet. It can be hard to not go along with the crowd. How have you been able to not take up smoking? What would you do if a friend tried to get you to smoke?" This line of questioning frames peer pressure as a potential influence on health.

Although being nonjudgmental is an important element of the medical interview, it is sometimes important to recognize that adolescents often wear their identity, literally, on their sleeve. That is, dress and physical appearance are common means for adolescents to make a statement about who they are or how they would like to be seen. For example, a 14-year-old boy was admitted to our adolescent medicine unit because of his refusal to eat, but he also refused to talk. When the attending physician entered the room, the boy was in his hospital bed wearing a knit cap pulled down to his eyebrows and ears, and an oversized T-shirt imprinted with the image of a television cartoon character. His pants were ¾-length oversized jeans with the crotch at midthigh and a heavy metal chain on the belt loop. His sneakers had flat, gum-rubber soles. After introducing himself, the physician asked the patient how he was doing and received no response. The next comment, "You look to me like a skateboarder," resulted in the patient establishing eye contact. The next question was, "Do you know any skateboard tricks?" The answer was "A few." This opened up a conversation about the patient's skateboarding, his friends, and things that he liked to do when he was "hanging out," which eventually led to a productive interview.

One should avoid overinterpreting the meaning of a teen's fashion or hair style. Not every youth who wears gang clothing or "colors" is a gang member.[10] However, one should not ignore the appearance of the adolescent being interviewed, especially if it seems incongruent with his or her background. Physical appearance often makes a statement about developing identity, but the message is not always clear. One needs to ask about these issues.

Cognitive Status

The transition from concrete to formal operations is a characteristic, although not universal, feature of adolescence. Concrete thinking is grounded in the here-and-now; abstract thinking enables the adolescent to think about thinking, hypothesize different explanations for an event, and suspend his or her own perceptions to consider the perceptions of others. If a patient has difficulty responding to questions, it may be because the patient is concrete operational. It also may be attributable to opposition, which may manifest in "closed" body language or facial expressions.

Egocentrism

Because the development of identity (ego) is central to adolescence, early-adolescent egocentrism is normal. In the medical interview, one can incorporate this by focusing on the adolescent as a person, not as a diagnosis or a problem. Similarly, the use of adjectival forms of diseases (epileptic) or disorders (bulimic) to describe a person should be avoided, because it is depersonalizing—exactly the opposite of egocentrism. In the interview, it is often better to frame the health problems as separate from who adolescents are as developing individuals with unique identities. They are not "bulimics," but "individuals who have bulimia."

Personal Fable

As adolescents gain a sense of mastery, they often assume a degree of invulnerability or invincibility, which can be seen in risky behaviors accompanied by an attitude of "nothing bad will happen to me." The interview can help determine if a teen's "risky" behavior is uninformed (unaware of the risks), risk-taking (defying limits), thrill-seeking (danger providing positive reinforcement), or normative activity to challenge one's self and learn one's own limits.

Imaginary Audience

The third element of adolescent cognitive changes that relates to the medical interview is the "imaginary audience," a construct in which early adolescents feel as if they are "on stage," with others thinking only about them. This can be considered as the intersection of egocentrism (in which the adolescent may view himself or herself as at the center of things) and formal operations (being able to think about abstractions such as thinking or taking another's viewpoint). However, the imaginary audience can interfere with the interview if the adolescent is self-absorbed while also being self-conscious about what the physician might be thinking about him or her. Strategies to lessen this negative influence include (1) use of screening questionnaires that shift the focus from what the adolescent might be thinking to what is written on the form,[11] (2) limiting pauses in the interview by maintaining conversational flow, and (3) including normalizing statements such as "I ask all of my patients your age about behaviors like substance use and sexual activity, because these can affect their health. Some, or all, of these questions may not apply to you. It lets you know that if you ever have any concerns in the future about anything that might affect your health, we can talk about them."

Box 1
Skills that underlie effective communication with adolescent patients

- Application of adolescent development principles
- Self-awareness
- Nonjudgmental approach
- Flexibility with consistency
- Active listening and observing

COMMUNICATION AS A KEY ELEMENT OF THE MEDICAL INTERVIEW

Skills That Facilitate Communication With Adolescents During the Medical Interview

There are abilities that underlie effective communication with adolescents (listed in Box 1).

Self-awareness

Whether the term "countertransference" or "gut reaction" is used, and whether it is negative or positive, an awareness of responses to the patient can facilitate communication being a shared process. In monitoring one's own responses, one may recognize that he or she is developing warm, empathetic feelings or is becoming anxious, bewildered, or angered by the topics being discussed. Patients often benefit from knowing their health care provider's views about issues, even if these views differ from their own. The critical issue in communicating is to share such information in a nonjudgmental manner.

Nonjudgmental Approach

The ability to react in a nonjudgmental manner is an essential communication skill for interviewing adolescents. Physicians are called on to make diagnostic, treatment, or prognostic judgments about illness and diseases. However, making value or moral judgments about the rightness or wrongness of behavior is generally nontherapeutic and can be countertherapeutic. A physician who has been personally affected by alcoholism may react strongly to an adolescent with a drinking problem; one opposed to premarital sex may wish to deny an adolescent's request for birth control pills on moral grounds. Such value-laden reactions may hinder an objective, therapeutic approach to the interview; instead of discussing health promotion, the teen is judged as a bad person, which impedes open communication. Being nonjudgmental does not mean that "anything goes" but, rather, requires an intermediate approach in which the interview serves to identify potential problems while showing acceptance of the adolescent as a person.

Flexibility With Consistency

In the medical interview, flexibility is the ability to adapt to new, unexpected, or unproductive situations and results in communication methods dictated by the patient and the problem(s) being addressed. It encourages the consideration of alternatives and options and models important healthy aspects of adult behavior. For example, a 14-year-old girl who had difficulty talking about her feelings with her therapist was sent to our clinic for additional evaluation. After introductions, the interviewer proceeded: "Let's start by talking about interesting things about you and your family, where you go to school, what you like to do with your friends, things like that. I'm going to ask you to keep a daily journal that you bring in with you on the next visit, and we can talk about what you've written there the next time we meet." Alternatively, reviewing a screening questionnaire could be useful, because it may be easier for an adolescent to endorse/deny symptoms rather than use language to describe his or her feelings.

Consistency in communication implies a certain predictability and stability that adolescents find reassuring. Consistent communication includes realistic limits and standards. When the adolescent exceeds those limits, for example, by using foul language, one can gently but firmly remind the adolescent, "Jon, in this clinic people respect each other. You are upset, and that's probably the way you talk to your parents at home. But foul language is not used here." Conversation could be resumed by saying, "Now, I was interested to hear you say that you don't think anyone listens to you at home. Can you tell me more about that?"

Active Listening and Observing

When used in conjunction with the skills listed above, the ability to actively listen and observe enables a physician to use information obtained in the interview. Being a listener and an observer that pursues understanding allows the interviewer to (1) listen to what is being said, how it is being said, and what is not being said, (2) observe the way the patient responds to questions, (3) obtain data from various sources, and (4) synthesize a unifying hypothesis to guide both the physical examination and treatment.

Techniques for Enhancing Adolescent Information-Sharing in the Medical Interview

In addition to the more abstract skills, there are specific techniques that can enhance adolescent engagement in the interview; these techniques are listed in Box 2 and are discussed below.

Engage the Patient as a Therapeutic Ally

For practitioners with a long-standing relationship with the patient, a therapeutic alliance may already exist. However, if there are ongoing struggles with parents,

Box 2
Techniques for enhancing adolescent information-sharing in the medical interview

- Engage the patient as a therapeutic ally
- Initiate the interview with nonthreatening topics
- Assume nothing
- Clarify inferences
- Provide confidentiality, but include patient in the collection of data from other sources
- Confront passive-aggressive behavior; substitute assertiveness
- Have the patient keep a daily journal
- Provide the patient with options from which to choose when discussing abstract concepts
- Link potentially embarrassing questions with health
- Use reflective responses
- Use summarizing statements
- Make use of body language

the patient may assume that the physician will take the side of his or her parents. If the adolescent appears to be resistant, it can be made explicit that many adolescents don't like coming to the doctor's office but that the physician will offer assistance in any way that will be helpful. At the outset, the physician establishes a position of neutral advocacy but makes use of the adolescent's normal egocentrism to build a therapeutic relationship.[12]

Initiate the Interview With Nonthreatening Topics

Although the traditional medical interview begins with the "chief complaint" and ends with a "problem list," identifying these elements at the beginning of the visit may not be helpful. To maintain a nonjudgmental posture, it is best to not define the patient's situation as a "problem" unless he or she is prepared to do so. By initiating the interview with conversation on relatively neutral issues such as hobbies, interests in music, sports, or likes and dislikes, one indirectly learns a great deal about an adolescent's behavior.

Assume Nothing

A physician should avoid assuming what an adolescent is thinking or feeling during the medical interview. Asking adolescents about their thoughts and feelings will not only facilitate communication about other health issues but also may help them to understand and express their emotions better by recognizing the link between emotions and health. Also, one should not make assumptions about the adolescent's sexual orientation or the gender of his or her sexual partner(s).

Clarify Inferences

Even when a patient's emotional state seems obvious, clarification should be sought to demonstrate empathy, stimulate discussion, and avoid misinterpretations. For example, a patient with school problems may become tearful when talking about her father's drinking problem but become embarrassed when she starts to cry and stop talking. Her tears might indicate sadness, anger at her father, disappointment with her grades, or fear that she will become an alcoholic. A response such as "You look upset" or "That seems to bother you" acknowledges the observed change in her emotional state and encourages her to talk further about her feelings.

Provide Confidentiality

As noted above, providing confidentiality and describing its limits and protections is one of the most important elements of the medical interview, especially with respect to adolescents who are engaged in behaviors typically addressed in state public health law provisions for confidential services.[13,14] This needs to be made explicit and may need to be repeated if the patient has denied such behavior but the data suggest otherwise.

Confront Passive-Aggressive Behavior; Substitute Assertiveness

Passive aggressiveness is characterized by passive behavior (forgetting, ignoring, delaying, etc) that channels hostility or aggressiveness (anger, frustration, violence) into socially acceptable acting out. It is a defensive maneuver encountered when an imbalance of power exists in a relationship, such as with a dominant physician versus a subordinate adolescent. The physician interviewing a passive-aggressive teen can confront the behavior in a calm and nonjudgmental manner but should be aware that denial is the usual response, possibly because of lack of awareness. The "I don't know" scenario noted earlier is a good example of passive aggressiveness. The key point is to not allow the behavior to frustrate one to the point of giving up, which only reinforces the behavior. Instead, it may be helpful to talk to the patient about the difference between aggressiveness and assertiveness. Assertiveness does not come naturally to a passive-aggressive adolescent, but it can be learned and, more importantly, role-modeled.

Have the Patient Keep a Daily Journal

A daily journal is a nonthreatening way for adolescents to record symptoms, emotions, and feelings and provides an insight into their daily life. Young adolescents may have neither the vocabulary nor the experience to express complex issues. A diary helps them develop, clarify, and organize their thoughts in a way that does not rely on verbal abilities or memory. It can also save time in the office, because the agenda for each visit can be the diary entries, obviating the need for an interim interview.

Provide the Patient With Options From Which to Choose When Discussing Abstract Concepts

Teens may need reassurance that they are normal. When their behavior is considered a problem, their normalcy is challenged. Prefacing queries with an emphasis on the wide range of normal can help: "Most of my patients who are having troubles such as yours don't like it. Some feel sad, some feel angry, some feel embarrassed, some feel guilty, and some feel picked on. How about you?" This lets the patient know that such feelings are normal. Teens may have difficulty describing emotions but can often deny or acknowledge having emotions in this manner.

Link Potentially Embarrassing Questions With Health

It is important to ask every adolescent about their health-risk behaviors, but for some adolescents the questions may be embarrassing or even offensive. It is important to inform all patients that the issues raised are discussed with all adolescents as part of comprehensive health supervision. Although the interviewer is often interested in identifying health-risk behaviors to be addressed, Ginsburg[15] and others have pointed out the importance of also engaging adolescents by building on their strengths.

Use Reflective Responses

A reflective response paraphrases the essence of statements made by the adolescent. It is not simply parroting whatever the adolescent says; it does not add any new content; it does not contain any bias; and it does not make any value judgments. A reflective response focuses selectively on what is judged to be the most important message in a statement made by an adolescent. It demonstrates active listening and observing and provides feedback to the adolescent about being understood. It also helps avoid detours in the interview process. For example, a 14-year-old boy was having difficulty controlling anger directed at his mother. He stated, "Sometimes I get so mad I think I am going to lose it. Like this morning when she hid the key to my bike. She had no right to do that. If she ever does that again, I won't be responsible for what happens." His mother responded, "Don't talk to me about rights; you have no rights when you act that way." To end this exchange, a physician could interrupt by putting his hand up, saying "Stop," and then noting to the teen, "Before you mentioned rights, you talked about getting mad. It sounds like you're concerned about losing control of your anger and having something bad happen. Tell me more about that."

Use Summarizing Statements

Especially useful when there are many symptoms or apparently disparate problem behaviors, synthesizing the key points into 1 or 2 summary concepts can help the patients, and parents, view organizing themes rather than a long list of problems. Mr Burns came to clinic with his son, Chris, and presented a full-page handwritten list of issues that he wanted to discuss. The son admitted remorsefully that he had taken the car on a few occasions and that he had a party while his parents were out of town. However, he thinks his parents judge his friends unfairly, so he lies when he goes out with them. He said fatalistically, "But they never believe anything I say, so I might as well take the blame for everything that goes wrong in our house." After hearing both sides of the story, the physician summarized the problem: "It seems like the main problem is one of trust, and neither one of you likes how things are going. Chris, you have shown some bad judgment recently, so your dad has reason to worry about trusting you. But, Mr Burns, it appears as if Chris is getting deeper and deeper into problems and thinks there is no way that he can ever can ever regain your trust. If this situation does not change, I suspect that the problems will only get worse. How can the two of you work on reestablishing a trusting father-son relationship?"

Make Use of Body Language

Although verbal communication is selectively intermittent and conscious, non-verbal communication is constant and often unconscious. Verbal communication gives an impression, while non-verbal communication creates an impression. Attending to nonverbal messages that are both transmitted and received can help a physician to be more effective in conducting the interview. Numerous nonverbal messages can acknowledge the special needs of adolescents, such as setting aside a few hours after school, in the evening, or on Saturday mornings to see adolescents and allowing at least 30 minutes for each visit. When a particularly difficult problem is identified during a routine visit, a follow-up visit can be scheduled at a more convenient time. As the patient gets older, more time is spent with the patient and less with the parents; by the time the patient is 15 or 16 years old, the patient can be seen alone for the entire visit. As previously noted, important body-language clues include dress, grooming, hair styling, facial expressions, eye contact, postures, gestures, and behaviors.

The interviewer communicates by means of body language as well: sitting with arms crossed or with the body held rigidly uptight or with the torso leaning away from the patient may convey a message of nonacceptance or being closed to communication. Not maintaining eye contact may cause the patient to infer that the physician is not interested, and glancing repeatedly at a watch or clock may send the message that time is being wasted. Taking extensive notes prevents eye contact and should be limited as much as possible. When it is necessary to take notes, either written or electronic, one can say, "I need to put down some facts to jog my memory later." Electronic medical charts can facilitate communication if the interviewer turns the screen so that the adolescent can also see what is being included. Body language can be used by a physician to facilitate communication in the interview: leaning toward the patient with one's hands naturally relaxed creates an impression of openness to talk about difficult issues, and at times of distress, light touches to the shoulder or hands can encourage talking, as can offering a tissue when a patient cries. Too-close contact may be threatening. Appropriate facial expressions to communicate concern, puzzlement, humor, and understanding indicate an interest in sharing open communication but should be well modulated.

TOOLS FOR STRUCTURING THE MEDICAL INTERVIEW WITH AN ADOLESCENT

Much of the information presented thus far does not have a specific structure but, rather, is based more on principles in the art of communicating with an adolescent. Developmental principles, skills, and techniques in the medical interview may be more regularly applied when the physician uses them within a structured visit. Structure provides scaffolding to the process that can help to keep the interviewer and the adolescent on task. Two examples of tools that provide structure to the interview will be discussed: screening questionnaires and mnemonics. Although such tools are generally used in the context of routine health supervision, rather than a visit to an emergency department or a specialty clinic, their elements can be used in any medical encounter.

Screening Questionnaires

A variety of screening questionnaires are available to identify health concerns in adolescents. The Guidelines for Adolescent Preventive Services (GAPS) form is perhaps the most widely used.[11] The health profile in the GAPS forms are especially time efficient, because the inner column of responses are the "positive" items that should be flagged for further discussion. A "no" response on the inner column for the item "Do you eat fruits and vegetables every day?" and a "yes" response in that same column for "Do you do things to lose weight (skip meals, take pills, starve yourself, vomit, etc)?" both deserve attention. An excerpt from the health profile section of the form for younger adolescents is shown in Fig 1.

Completion of such a form (either on paper or electronically) before a visit requires the patient to think about issues that might be addressed and ensures that a comprehensive screening survey is in the record. It also provides a rapid means to identify areas that require further discussion.

Mnemonics

In the absence of a written or computerized screening instrument, mnemonics are useful clinical tools to remind clinicians about things to include when developing differential diagnoses, considering the causes of symptoms or signs, or asking patients questions during a clinical interview. A limitation of most mnemonics is their lack of active involvement of the adolescent; they are anagrams that assist

Guidelines for Adolescent Preventive Services
Younger Adolescent Questionnaire (excerpt)

Health Profile

Eating/Weight/Body
14. Do you eat fruits and vegetables every day? .... ☐ No ☐ Yes
15. Do you drink milk and/or eat milk products every day? .... ☐ No ☐ Yes
16. Do you spend a lot of time thinking about ways to be skinny? .... ☐ Yes ☐ No
17. Do you do things to lose weight (skip meals, take pills, starve yourself, vomit, etc) .... ☐ Yes ☐ No
18. Do you work, play, or exercise enough to make you sweat or breathe hard at least 3 times a week? .... ☐ No ☐ Yes
19. Have you pierced your body (not including ears) or gotten a tattoo? .... ☐ No ☐ Yes

Fig 1. The Guidelines for Adolescent Preventive Services younger-adolescent questionnaire (excerpt).

the clinician and may not engage or teach patients. A popular mnemonic in adolescent health care is HEADS, a psychosocial risk assessment instrument that was later modified by Cohen et al[16] to include an additional "S" (ie, HEADSS) at the end. The interview starts by asking about home, then education and employment, followed by questions about activities, drugs, sexuality, and suicide/depression. These topics cover the majority of issues to be discussed in psychosocial risk assessment but do not focus on pertinent items such as family medical history or strengths of the adolescent.

The mnemonic PACES, used to facilitate interviewing adolescents for comprehensive health supervision, has several advantages because it (1) places the adolescent in the context of his or her environment, (2) includes a family history, (3) has a logical flow from general to specific, (4) engages the adolescent in the process of thinking about relevant causes of morbidity and mortality by a highly Socratic method, (5) facilitates discussion and open communication about a wide variety of strategies for avoiding or minimizing health problems, (6) provides opportunities to emphasize strengths and health-promoting behaviors, (7) offers an opportunity to educate adolescents at "teachable moments," and (8) prepares the adolescent to be an adult consumer of health care. A clinical scenario using PACES follows.

"Teri, it's good to see you. Now that you are an adolescent, there are different things that you need to be thinking about to keep yourself healthy. You are no longer a child, but not yet an adult. To remind myself of the questions I want to ask all of my teenaged patients, I use the word 'PACES' because each letter stands for something that can affect their health. Are you ready to go through the PACES for your health?"

"The 'P' in PACES stands for 'peers' and 'parents.' First, we'll start with peers, because if your peers have some health problems, you may have them, too. What do you think are the main health problems for your peers, people your age, your friends?" [Wait for an answer. If no answer, probe for what might cause kids to get sick or be hospitalized or die. Then, ask if those things have happened to any of his or her friends or classmates. Whatever the answer is, the goal is to work from the peer group to the individual adolescent with whom you are speaking.] "Have you ever had any of those things?" [If no, you can ask what he or she has done to prevent them. If yes, explore them, but only briefly. You do not want to get bogged down in an in-depth clinical interview. The purpose of putting an adolescent through the PACES is to screen for conditions.]

"The 'P' is also for 'parents.' How is your father's health? How about your mother's health? Do either of them take medicines or need to see the doctor often? Do they have any habits that make you worry about their health? [This encourages exploration of habits such as eating, smoking, drinking alcohol, or using other substances and is better than asking, "Is your father an alcoholic?"] How about other family members, like your brothers or sisters? Are your grandparents still alive? [The purpose is not to perform an exhaustive family history but to get a sense of the patient's family context. If there is a family history of a parent taking a cholesterol-lowering drug or having been hospitalized, this can be addressed after going through the PACES by saying, "I want to get back to that after going through the PACES."]

"The 'A' in PACES stands for the major cause of death for young people your age. What do you think that is?" [This Socratic technique is used to engage the adolescent patient in the encounter and to get him or her thinking about health-related behaviors. The correct answer is "accidents," but if he or she answers "alcohol," that is also correct, because at least half of motor vehicle accidents are related to alcohol use. If the adolescent answers either of these questions, affirm the response to keep him or her engaged. If he or she gives an answer such as "cancer," which does not begin with an "a," you can respond with an encouraging negative like, "That's what a lot of people think, but it doesn't begin with an 'a,' like 'accidents' does. That's the leading cause of death for young people your age, and about half of accidents are related to another 'a,' alcohol use."] "Have any of your friends (or you) ever had an accident? What do they (or you) do to prevent accidents?" [This also allows you to make the questioning developmentally appropriate. A 14-year-old needs to be wearing protective gear when he or she is skateboarding, a 15-year-old needs to wear a seat-belt every time he or she gets into a car, and a 16-year-old needs to not get into a car in which the driver is intoxicated. This also allows you to tailor the questioning to the environment. For example, if the adolescent is from a neighborhood marked by violence, accidents can be reframed in terms of "assault." The concept of accidents is broad, and the flexibility of PACES allows you to respond to individual situations.]

"The 'C' in PACES stands for the leading 'cause' of sickness and death among adults but is a habit that usually starts before age 18. What do you think that might be?" [The correct answer is smoking cigarettes. When the patient says this, give a very positive "yes" to keep him or her engaged. Depending on the clinical situation, this may need to be expanded to other tobacco products such as cigars, snuff, or chew, although these products are much less likely to be used than cigarettes, especially by females. If he or she answers "cancer," you can respond with an encouraging negative like noted above: "In a way, that's right, because a lot of cancer is caused by cigarettes, but cigarettes also cause lots of other illness besides cancer."] "How many of your friends smoke?" [This may already have been addressed with the peer health question at the beginning of PACES, so you may need to adapt.] "How much do you smoke?" [If the adolescent appears offended that you might think he or she smokes, provide positive encouragement such as, "When so many kids your age are smoking, how have you avoided it?" or "It sounds like you choose your friends pretty carefully and don't hang around with anyone who smokes. That's great, because who you hang around with can affect your health."] "What would you do if someone came up to you and offered you a cigarette? What would you do?" [This also provides an opportunity to provide positive reinforcement for appropriate responses such as, "I'd just say, 'no thanks,' and walk away." If the adolescent is a smoker, this also provides an opportunity to advise him or her to stop smoking, assist in the attempt to stop smoking if desired, and arrange for follow-up.]

"The 'E' in PACES stands for a lot of things. Can you think of something that begins with the letter 'e' that can affect your health, either good or bad"? [Items that begin with the letter "e" that should be explored include exercise, eating, and emotions. The physician can continue using the same kind of Socratic method in each of these areas to keep the patient engaged. Positive behaviors with respect to any of these domains should be reinforced as a strength-building technique. Some adolescents may not make the link between emotions but this can be facilitated by the query, "What do you think is the second leading cause of death for kids your age, after car crashes?" The answer is suicide, and the link between emotions and suicide are usually well understood. This also provides an opportunity to inquire about what the adolescent would do if a friend told him or her about being suicidal; a good answer is, "Tell an adult whom you trust."]

"Finally, the 'S' in PACES stands for 'school' and 'sexuality.' You probably know some ways in which sexual activity can affect an adolescent's health, but school is also related to health. It helps to do well in school if you are healthy, and teens who are not in school sometimes aren't as healthy as those who are." [Using the kind of probes mentioned in the other elements of the PACES format can help to place these domains in the context of health and provide an opportunity to reinforce health-promoting behaviors and discuss strategies for reducing risk.]

CONCLUSIONS

This article provides both theoretical and practical considerations to help guide the physician while conducting a medical interview in the context of evaluation and management in adolescent medicine. Focusing on each adolescent as an individual who is progressing from childhood to adulthood, with development tasks to accomplish, helps to frame key areas for attention. Applying the skills and techniques detailed, as well as using screening tools and mnemonics, can aid the physician in engaging the adolescent in a process that is sufficiently structured, goal oriented, and productive to make the medical interview enjoyable for both parties. Not mentioned, however, is "the secret" to the medical interview that was identified by Peabody[16] almost 80 years ago: "the secret of the care of the patient is in caring for the patient."

REFERENCES

1. Stickler GB. Are yearly physical examinations in adolescents necessary? *J Am Board Fam Pract.* 2000;13(3):172–177
2. Elster AB. Comparison of recommendations for adolescent clinical preventive services developed by national organizations. *Arch Pediatr Adolesc Med.* 1998;152(2):193–198
3. Roberts TA, Auinger P, Ryan SA. Body piercing and high-risk behavior in adolescents. *J Adolesc Health.* 2004;34(3):224–229
4. Steinberg L. *Adolescence.* 8th ed. New York, NY: McGraw-Hill; 2007
5. Gilligan C. *In a Different Voice: Psychological Theory and Women's Development.* Cambridge, MA: Harvard University Press; 1982
6. Klein JD, Hedberg VA, Allan M, Flatau C. Do providers and adolescents agree about confidentiality? *J Adolesc Health.* 1996;18(2):151
7. Thrall JS, McCloskey L, Rothstein E, et al. Perception of confidentiality and adolescents' use of health care services and information. *J Adolesc Health.* 1997;20(2):163
8. Lehrer JA, Pantell R, Tebb K, Shafer MA. Forgone health care among U.S. adolescents: associations between risk characteristics and confidentiality concern, 14 December 2006. *J Adolesc Health.* 2007;40(3):218–226
9. Ford CA, Thomsen SL, Compton B. Adolescents' interpretations of conditional confidentiality assurances. *J Adolesc Health.* 2001;29(3):156–159
10. Institute for Intergovernmental Research. National Youth Gang Center. Available at: www.iir.com/NYGC. Accessed September 1, 2007
11. Gadomski A, Bennett S, Young M, Wissow LS. Guidelines for Adolescent Preventive Services: the GAPS in practice. *Arch Pediatr Adolesc Med.* 2003;157(5):426–432
12. Ryan RM, Deci EL. Autonomy is no illusion: self-determination theory and the empirical study of authenticity, awareness, and will. In: Greenberg J, Koole S, Pyszczynski T, eds. *Handbook of Experimental Existential Psychology.* New York, NY: Guilford; 2004: 449–479
13. Morreale MC, Stinnett AJ, Dowling EC. Policy compendium on confidential health services for adolescents: second edition (2005). Available at: www.cahl.org/PolicyCompendium.htm. Accessed September 1, 2007
14. English A, Kenny KE. State minor consent laws: a summary—second edition (2003). Available at: www.cahl.org/MC%20Monograph.htm. Accessed September 1, 2007
15. McClain B. Building resilience in children. Available at: www.aap.org/family/healthychildren/07winter/bldgresil.pdf. Accessed September 1, 2007
16. Peabody FW. Landmark article March 19, 1927: The care of the patient. *JAMA.* 1984;252(6):813–818

Interviewing the Adolescent With an Eating Disorder

Cathleen Steinegger, MD,
Debra K. Katzman, MD, FRCP(C)*

Division of Adolescent Medicine, and Department of Pediatrics, Hospital for Sick Children and University of Toronto, 555 University Avenue, Toronto, Ontario, Canada M5G 1X8

Interviewing an adolescent is a fundamental component of the overall assessment of an adolescent with an eating disorder (Tables 1–3).[1] The interview helps to establish the diagnosis, risk factors, comorbidities, medical complications, and initial treatment plan.[2,3] If done in a thoughtful and compassionate manner, the interview can establish the foundation of a therapeutic alliance among the clinician, the adolescent, and her family.

Because the majority of adolescents with eating disorders are female, we refer to adolescents in this article as female; the interview would have the same format and content (excluding the menstrual history) regardless of the gender of the patient.

THE CHALLENGES OF INTERVIEWING AN ADOLESCENT WITH AN EATING DISORDER

Interviewing an adolescent with an eating disorder can be challenging for many reasons. Adolescents with eating disorders often minimizes or denies her symptoms. This is attributable, in part, to her distorted perception of the facts but may also be an effort to keep the clinician from knowing about her eating-disordered behaviors so that she can continue them. If the adolescent denies having a problem, the clinician can express that he or she is concerned about what the adolescent is communicating, worried about the adolescent's health and well-being, and reassured that the adolescent is in the clinician's office for an evaluation.

Adolescents may not perceive themselves as having a problem with food, because disordered eating behaviors may be common among their peers. Alter-

*Corresponding author.
E-mail address: debra.katzman@sickkids.ca (D. K. Katzman).

Copyright © 2008 American Academy of Pediatrics. All rights reserved. ISSN 1934-4287

Table 1
DSM-IV criteria for anorexia nervosa

Refusal to maintain body weight above 85% of that expected for gender, age, and height or failure to make expected weight gain during period of growth, leading to body weight below 85% of that expected

Intense fear of gaining weight or becoming fat, even though underweight

Disturbance in the way in which one's body weight, size, or shape is experienced, undue influence of body weight or shape on self-evaluation, or denial of the seriousness of the current low body weight

In postmenarcheal females, absence of at least three consecutive menstrual cycles when otherwise expected to occur (primary or secondary amenorrhea)

Two subtypes of anorexia nervosa are defined: restrictive type (during the current episode, the person has not regularly engaged in binge eating or purging behavior) and binge-purge type (during the current episode, the person has regularly engaged in binge eating or purging behavior).

natively, adolescents may be embarrassed and humiliated by their eating attitudes and behaviors and, therefore, find them difficult to discuss, particularly if they do not know their clinician well. Therefore, adolescents with eating disorders rarely refer themselves for assessment or treatment. The referral is often made by the adults in their lives.

Eating disorders can develop at any time during adolescence.[4,5] As such, the unique physical, cognitive, and social developmental processes of adolescence may result in some adolescents who lack understanding or self-awareness with respect to body shape, weight, or size and, therefore, may not be able to answer certain questions.

Table 2
DSM-IV criteria for bulimia nervosa

Recurrent episodes of binge eating; an episode of binge eating is characterized by both of the following:
  Eating, in a discrete period of time (eg, within any 2-h period), an amount of food that is definitely larger than most people would eat during a similar period of time and under similar circumstances
  A sense of lack of control over eating during the episode
Recurrent inappropriate compensatory behavior to prevent weight gain, such as self-induced vomiting; misuse of laxatives, diuretics, enemas, or other medications; fasting; or excessive exercise
The binge eating and inappropriate compensatory behaviors both occur, on average, at least twice per week for 3 mo
Self-evaluation is unduly influenced by body shape and weight
The disturbance does not occur exclusively during episodes of anorexia nervosa

---

Two subtypes are defined: purging type (during the current episode of bulimia nervosa, the person has regularly engaged in self-induced vomiting or the misuse of laxative, diuretics, or enemas) and nonpurging type (during the current episode of bulimia nervosa, the person has used other inappropriate compensatory behaviors such as fasting or excessive exercise but has not regularly engaged in self-induced vomiting or the misuse of laxative, diuretics, or enemas).

Table 3
DSM-IV criteria for eating disorder, not otherwise specified

For females, all of the criteria for anorexia nervosa are met except that the individual has regular menses

All of the criteria for anorexia nervosa are met except that, despite significant weight loss, the individual's current weight is >85% of a healthy weight

All of the criteria for bulimia nervosa are met except that the binge eating and inappropriate compensatory mechanisms occur at a frequency of less than twice per week or for a duration of <3 mo

The regular use of inappropriate compensatory behavior by an individual of normal body weight after eating small amounts of food

Repeatedly chewing and spitting out, not swallowing, large amounts of food

Binge-eating disorder: recurrent episodes of binge eating in the absence of the regular use of inappropriate compensatory behaviors that are characteristic of bulimia nervosa

Adolescents with eating disorders may be acutely aware of the stigma associated with eating disorders. Some adolescents may be concerned about being labeled or criticized. Furthermore, adolescents with eating disorders may be afraid that asking for help will result in loss of control over their lives. Despite these challenges, clinicians with a solid understanding of adolescent behavior in general, and eating disorders in particular, can develop interview techniques that will overcome these hurdles. Acknowledging these barriers in the interview will often help put the adolescent at ease despite the anxiety of the situation.

As a result of the barriers outlined above, the clinician should be prepared for the possibility that the adolescent will not necessarily arrive at an assessment knowingly or willingly and may be very angry about the process. An example of such a situation is the adolescent who has been told by her concerned parent(s)/guardian(s) that they have made an appointment for her to see the clinician because she "has not had her menstrual period for the past 6 months," only to be informed in the waiting room (or in an examination room by the clinician) that she is there for an eating disorder assessment. Under such circumstances, it is not surprising that the adolescent may be angry and choose to avoid conversation about her eating attitudes and behaviors. It is important to talk openly with the adolescent about this situation and acknowledge the reasons for her feelings.

APPROACHING THE INTERVIEW

Imagine the adolescent and family in the waiting room. The adolescent may be angry, embarrassed, and humiliated. The parent(s)/guardian(s) are concerned, worried, and remorseful. The clinician should be approachable and direct, providing a clear description and outline of what is going to happen during the assessment.

There are many ways to structure an interview with an adolescent and her family. The clinician can meet with the adolescent alone first. This approach can give the adolescent the message that she is the clinician's patient and that the clinician is most eager to hear what the patient has to say. On the other hand, the clinician can choose to meet with the adolescent and her parent(s)/guardian(s) together for the initial part of the interview and then meet with the adolescent alone. We have found the latter approach very helpful for a number of reasons. This approach allows the clinician to communicate that he or she values input from both the adolescent and her parent(s) and that he or she regards the parent(s)/guardian(s) as an important support for the adolescent while she is recovering from an eating disorder.[6] With the adolescent present, the clinician can acknowledge the worry and concern expressed by most parent(s)/guardian(s) of an adolescent who shows signs and symptoms of an eating disorder. It can also be very helpful for the adolescent to hear her parent(s)/guardian(s) express their concerns. This approach also provides a way for the clinician to observe the dynamics of the relationship between the adolescent and her parent(s)/guardian(s). How an adolescent relates to her parent(s)/guardian(s) during the interview provides a wealth of information. Where does the adolescent sit in relation to one or both parent(s)/guardian(s)? Is the adolescent-parent connection characterized by warmth, kindness, and respect? Does the adolescent listen to and hear what the parent(s)/guardian(s) are saying? Does the parent(s)/guardian(s) listen to and hear what the adolescent is saying? Does the adolescent verbally respond to questions in the presence of the parent(s)/guardian(s), or does she roll her eyes, shrug her shoulders, or leave the room? Does the adolescent respond to their concerns with compassion or anger?

CONFIDENTIALITY

Regardless of the interview structure, an open discussion about confidentiality and the limits of confidentiality should be reviewed with the adolescent and her parent(s)/guardian(s). The legal definition of confidentiality will vary depending on the geographic location. It is the responsibility of clinicians to familiarize themselves with the legal issues of confidentiality in their locality. The clinician should articulate what he or she can and cannot keep confidential. With this information, the adolescent can make a choice about how much to reveal during the interview. Although the adolescent may not provide the clinician with a lot of information on the first meeting, adolescents are more willing to disclose sensitive information to clinicians who give assurances of confidentiality.[7]

Here is one way to approach to the concept of confidentiality with the adolescent and her parent(s)/guardian(s): "Before we start, I wanted to let you know about how confidentiality works in my clinic. Whatever Beth tells me today during this interview is confidential—that means that it is private between me and Beth. I'm not allowed to discuss the interview with you [parent(s)/guardian(s)] without Beth's permission. However, there are some important exceptions. For example, if Beth tells me something that makes it clear that either Beth or others are at 'significant health risk or harm,' then I would inform you. Beth, if you're not sure whether you or someone is at 'significant health risk or harm,' why don't you ask me before answering the question?"

For a case in which the clinician works as part of a team, he or she might add, "Lastly, all of you need to know that I will be sharing what we talk about with the other members of the assessment team."

Finally, remember to invite the adolescent and her parent(s)/guardian(s) to ask questions at any time during the interview.

GETTING STARTED

With the adolescent and her parent(s)/guardian(s) together, the clinician can determine who made the appointment and why, who is concerned about the adolescent, and which behaviors or attitudes are the source of their concern. Once the clinician has accomplished this, he or she can request to meet with the adolescent alone: "Thanks Mr and Mrs Smith. You have been very helpful. Now, I would like to meet with Beth alone. There may be questions that arise or concerns that you have that you would like to discuss. Please keep track of these things so that we can address them. Please have a seat in the waiting room, and I will invite you back to join me and Beth after we [Beth and the clinician] have had a chance to talk."

The initial contact with the adolescent will set the tone for the interview. The clinician's primary goals will be to understand the reason(s) for referral, establish confidentiality, and start to develop a therapeutic alliance. It is important to convey empathy, interest, understanding, honesty, and support while avoiding judgmental or critical attitudes and undue familiarity. The clinician should pay careful attention to his or her tone of voice, words, and body language. He or she should make an effort to be sensitive about the way he or she addresses the adolescent with an eating disorder. Inadvertently, the clinician may say things that are harmful or misinterpreted by the adolescent. Some of these things include oversimplifying the eating disorder or judging the adolescent's behaviors and feelings (Table 4). Furthermore, the clinician should be aware of his or her attitudes about his or her own weight and shape and that of others, including the patient's.

Adolescents who are referred for an evaluation for an eating disorder will present at varying physical, cognitive, and social developmental stages. When conducting an interview, the clinician should be mindful of the adolescent's age and developmental stage. Early adolescents are concrete thinkers and have limited abilities to understand abstract thoughts. As the adolescent matures, she will develop the ability to think more abstractly, use logic, and see and understand things from multiple perspectives.[8] The clinician should attempt to communicate with the adolescent at her developmental stage.

Table 4
What not to say to an adolescent with an eating disorder

What the Clinician Says	What the Adolescent With an Eating Disorder Thinks
"You look great!"	"I am so fat!"
"It is great that you got your menstrual period."	"Oh no, I must be fat!"
"I am so pleased that you ate the WHOLE chocolate bar."	"Oh no, I am out of control."
"You've gained 2 lb over the last week … looks like you're gaining a little too quickly."	Better start restricting my intake, I'm obviously getting fat."
"Now that you've put on a few pounds, you're looking more like your sister."	"My 9-year-old sister has so much baby fat! That is disgusting."
"Your face is getting full."	"My body is so huge!"
"From the sounds of your daily intake, you are eating a lot better."	"How could I consume all the food?"
"Now that you've reached your ideal body weight, you can start eating healthy again."	"Yes, I can start eating celery, carrot sticks, and low-fat yogurt."
"If you'd just eat normally, things would be fine."	"As if it is that simple! I wish the doctor would understand how difficult this is for me and how much I want to stop binging and purging! I can't stand doing these things and I can't stand feeling this way!"
"All you have to do is accept yourself as you are."	"I can't stand myself; how could I possibly accept myself?"
"Even though you are binging and purging, I am not as concerned about you now that you are at a normal weight."	"The doctor thinks because I'm at a normal weight that I am not sick enough; well, maybe I should lose some more weight."

Creating a respectful relationship with the adolescent is important to the success of the interview. The establishment of the therapeutic alliance is one of the major tasks and challenges faced by the clinician. The therapeutic alliance is created by providing a safe, nonjudgmental environment in which the adolescent feels that she can talk openly about her thoughts and feelings. Several interview techniques facilitate this process and include expressing empathy to the adolescent ("That sounds very upsetting…"), acknowledging her feelings ("I see that you are upset by this…."), reviewing what she has said and clarifying that the clinician understands ("This is what I'm hearing you say…. Is that correct?"), and shedding light on her behaviors ("Other adolescents with eating problems have told me they…. Have you ever done that?"). More examples of how to use these strategies to build rapport are discussed below.

Although some adolescents come to an eating-disorder assessment planning to avoid any discussion around eating, the clinician's ability to demonstrate a clear grasp of the adolescent's personal experience with an eating disorder will increase the adolescent's willingness to engage in a discussion about her disorder.

IDENTIFYING THE PROBLEM

Start off the questioning by exploring the reasons why the adolescent has come to the clinic; clinicians should not assume that they know the reasons. Adolescents arrive at their eating-disorder assessment with a variety of feelings that range from relief that they are going to get help to denial of any problem with eating. It is helpful to find out from the outset where the adolescent is along this continuum so that the clinician can approach the interview appropriately. One might say, "Adolescents who come to their doctor for troubles with eating have many different feelings about the visit. Some have been 'dragged here' because either their parents or someone else believes that there is a problem with the young person's eating, weight, or feelings about their body. Others recognize that they are struggling with these issues and want to be here. Many sit somewhere between. Where do you see yourself in terms of there being a problem with your eating, weight, or body image?" If the adolescent has trouble with this question, it may be helpful to have her rank herself on a scale from 1 to 10, with "1" meaning she feels she has absolutely no problem with eating and "10" meaning she has a terrible problem and needs to be hospitalized. If her parent(s)/guardian(s) are still in the room, it may be useful to have them rank their daughter's problems with eating on the same scale. This is a simple way to get everyone's thoughts about the situation out in the open.

Unless the adolescent has answered that she believes she has absolutely no problem with eating, the next question should be, "What do you think the problem is?" followed by, "What do you think the solution is?" These questions help build rapport by indicating to the adolescent that her clinician cares about her opinion and wants her to be part of the treatment team. If possible, the clinician should try to refer back to her answers to these questions later in the interview so that the adolescent knows that he or she was truly listening. Even if a clearly emaciated adolescent says her problem is that she is "too fat," one can say, "I am hearing that you feel this way. Many adolescents with eating disorders feel this way, even when it is not true from a medical/health point of view. One of our goals will be to help you deal with this feeling in a way that does not harm your health." If the adolescent does not believe that she has any problems with eating, the clinician may proceed to ask the parent(s)/guardian(s) what they see as the problem behavior and what kind of help they are hoping to get for their daughter.

WEIGHT HISTORY

After inquiring about the presenting problem, more historical information should be obtained. This may be prefaced with, "I am going to be asking you some specific questions about your eating behaviors and feelings so that I can get a better understanding of what it's like for you." Ask questions to get a clear picture of the evolution of her illness. How and when did it start? Was she trying to lose weight and, if yes, why? What were her initial attempts at weight control? Did this work? How did her symptoms progress? How much weight did she lose? Over what length of time? When and why did she or others become concerned about her eating behaviors? Determine if the adolescent has ever been teased about her body weight, shape, or size.[9] Abnormal eating attitudes and behaviors may occur after a comment about one's appearance by a family member, teacher, coach, health care provider, or peer. Triggering events may be identified by asking, "What happened? Did anything specific occur around that time, or did someone say something that made you focus on your shape or weight?" Later in treatment, it may be helpful to look back at the triggering events with the adolescent and identify other ways to cope with these challenging situations. Finally, the question "How did people respond to your change in weight?" may identify perpetuating or protective factors. It is not uncommon for an adolescent who has lost weight to initially be praised for "looking good" or "getting healthy" and to have this positive reinforcement strengthen the adolescent's commitment to further weight loss. On the other hand, concerns voiced by others about the weight loss and other physical changes may help the adolescent realize that she has a problem and motivate her to consider change.

An accurate weight history is crucial when making the diagnosis and determining the severity of an eating disorder. It also helps to establish the therapeutic goal weight for the adolescent. Ideally, this is an adolescent whom the clinician has followed for many years and, therefore, will have a well-maintained growth chart. If not, it is helpful to get previous weight and height information to establish the adolescent's premorbid growth pattern.

The clinician should ask the adolescent about her past highest and lowest weights, when these weights occurred, and for how long. If the adolescent has secondary amenorrhea, the clinician will want to know the weight at which she lost her menstrual period. This is one of a number of clinical factors that might be helpful when determining a minimum goal weight associated with the return of menstrual function.[10] Exploring the disparity between what the adolescent understands her healthy weight to be (ie, the weight she thinks a doctor would want her to be) and what she wants her weight to be, will give the clinician a sense of the adolescent's knowledge about healthy weight and if she can apply this knowledge to herself.

DIETARY HISTORY

A detailed dietary history is helpful when making a diagnosis and recognizing the potential medical complications. Having the adolescent describe a typical day of eating will establish the adolescent's energy intake and eating attitudes and behaviors. A 24-hour dietary recall, including types of foods and beverages consumed and portion sizes, can highlight whether the diet is adequate, balanced, and structured. Adolescents with eating disorders may consume a large quantity of diet products and may avoid fats and carbohydrates. They may also drink an excessive amount of fluids including caffeinated products such as coffee, tea, or diet soda to reduce hunger and alter body weight. The adolescent may need prompts to provide important details. For example:

> Clinician: "It would really help me if you described what you eat on a typical school day. Why don't we just walk through the day . . . let's start with what time you usually wake up."
>
> Adolescent: "6 o'clock."
>
> Clinician: "Tell me how your day begins, starting with the first time you have something to eat."
>
> Adolescent: "After getting ready for school, I have my breakfast."
>
> Clinician: "Do you have breakfast with your family?"
>
> Adolescent: "No."
>
> Clinician: "Do you have breakfast by yourself?"
>
> Adolescent. "My dad leaves for work early in the morning and my mom is in the shower. My brother is still asleep. So, I eat by myself."
>
> Clinician: "So do you prepare your breakfast?"
>
> Adolescent: "Yes."
>
> Clinician: "What do you have for breakfast?"
>
> Adolescent: "Cereal."
>
> Clinician: "How much cereal, and what kind?"
>
> Adolescent: "Usually a small bowl of bran flakes."
>
> Clinician: "If I were to measure a 'small bowl,' would that be a half cup or 1 cup?"
>
> Adolescent: "I measure it out, and it is always a cup. That's 1 serving on the label."

Clinician: "Do you have milk on the cereal?"

Adolescent: "Yes."

Clinician: "What kind of milk?"

Adolescent: "Skim milk."

Clinician: "How much skim milk?"

Adolescent: "I measure 1 cup of skim milk."

Clinician: "Okay, so for breakfast you have 1 cup of bran flakes with skim milk. Anything else?"

Adolescent: "No, that's it."

Clinician. "All right. Thanks for the details. Now, let's move on to the next time in a day when you have something to eat . . . ."

This should continue until a daily schedule of eating has been completed. As can be seen from this sample dialogue, the clinician often has to do quite a lot of prompting and exploring to get the specific dietary details. Most adolescents are acutely aware of exactly what they eat (many are writing it down in detail) and, with prompting, will provide the clinician with an extremely accurate representation of their intake, including exactly how many calories and grams of fat they consume per day.

This is an opportune time to get an understanding from the adolescent about her family's attitudes and behaviors about food, weight loss, and health. What are meal times like? Does she participate in family meals, or does she eat alone? If she eats alone, why? Who does the grocery shopping? Who prepares meals? What types of food does her family eat? Is there a lot of talk about "health," "dieting," or "exercise" at home?

EATING-DISORDER BEHAVIORS

There are multiple unhealthy techniques used by adolescents with eating disorders to control their weight (listed in Table 5 along with sample questions). The clinician should ask about each of these methods separately and probe for specific details. It is important to let the adolescent know that these methods are ineffective and dangerous. One way to preface these questions is to say, "I'm going to be asking you about different ways that young people use to try to control their weight and body shape. Before I do, I want you to know that there is medical research that tells us that these methods are ineffective. You also need to know that all these methods can be extremely dangerous. Many young people believe these methods work, but they

Table 5
Weight-control measures

General questions
  "How do you feel about your weight?"
  "Have you had a recent change in your weight?"
  "What have you done to change your weight or body shape?"
  "Are you afraid of gaining weight or being overweight?"
  "Have you had a menstrual period?" If yes, "When was your last menstrual period?"
Fasting
  "Have you ever tried to go for a long period of time without eating anything?"
  "For how long would you do that?"
  "When was the last time you did this?"
  "How typical has that been for you over the past week/month?"
  "Do you have any thoughts about what causes you to do this?"
Binging
  "Do you ever eat an amount of food that is larger than what other young people your age would eat?"
  "Do you ever feel that your eating is out of control or that you are powerless to stop eating?"
  "Are there times when you can't stop eating even when you are full?"
  "Are there certain things that "set you off" like being stressed, upset, or angry that causes you to binge?"
Self-induced vomiting
  "Do you ever vomit to keep yourself from gaining weight?"
  "How often in the last month?"
  "Are there certain things that 'set you off,' such as being stressed, upset, or angry, that cause you to vomit?
  "How do you make yourself vomit (fingers, spoon, automatic, etc)?"
  "Have you ever vomited blood?"
Medication and substance use
  "Do you ever use laxatives, diuretics, ipecac, diet pills, other medications, complementary or alternative medications, or other supplements to keep yourself from gaining weight?"
  "How often do you take them?"
  "How many at one time?"
  "Have you ever experienced a side effect or unpleasant consequence from taking these things?"
Excessive exercise
  "What kind do you do?"
  "How long at one time?"
  "How many times per day? Per week?"
  "Do you exercise alone or with others?"
  "Do you ever force yourself to exercise, even if you don't want to or when you are injured?"
  "Do you ever get upset if you miss a workout or can't exercise?"
  "Do you primarily exercise to influence your weight and body shape?"

---

don't. Please feel free to ask me about any of these methods and we can talk about it more." Inviting questions from the adolescent helps to decrease her shame and opens up an opportunity for education.

Food Restriction

An adolescent with an eating disorder will often restrict her diet to a minimal number of calories and a few types of low fat foods. One can elicit this information by determining the adolescent's caloric intake on the basis of her 24-hour dietary recall and asking, "Are there any foods that you avoid?" If the answer is yes, then ask, "Why? Do you have 'good (or safe)' or 'bad (or unsafe)' foods? Can you give me examples of 'good' or 'bad' foods? What foods do you feel most safe eating? Do you ever hide or throw away food?" It is also important to ask about vegetarianism, because this is common among adolescents with eating disorders. Ask why the adolescent is or has become a vegetarian (religious, ethical, or weight-loss reasons). Is this part of the eating disorder or is this an individual or shared family value?[11]

Food Rituals

Some adolescents with eating disorders develop food rituals, often as a way to slow down, delay, or avoid eating at all. They may be embarrassed about these rituals, so it helps to demystify the behaviors before asking the questions: "Some adolescents with eating problems, especially if they are trying to eat a small amount of food, develop habits or rituals around eating that others may find unusual. For example, some cut their food into a certain number of pieces, or chew each bite a specific number of times. Do you do anything like this?" Other examples of food rituals include using tiny utensils, eating food in a certain order, and only eating foods of a particular color. Foods previously enjoyed by the adolescent are often avoided. Adolescents with eating disorders tend to eat the same foods at the same time each day. These behaviors are often confused with obsessive-compulsive disorder but usually disappear with normalization of nutritional intake and weight rehabilitation.

It is not uncommon for adolescents with eating disorders to develop a strong interest in shopping for food, cooking for others, reading cookbooks, and watching food-related programs on television. Parent(s)/guardians will report that they can't believe their daughter has a problem with food because "she cooks for us all the time!" They may not realize that although she is cooking for everyone else, she is not eating any of the food she has prepared.

Exercise

It is important to explore the adolescent's exercise history. Does the adolescent exercise, and if so, what type of exercise? Why does she exercise? How often and for how long? Does she participate in group exercise activities or "work out" by herself? Does the adolescent participate in sport or dance training that requires long hours of practice or focuses on body shape, weight, and size? The specifics are important, as illustrated below:

> Clinician: "What kinds of exercise do you and your friends do for fun?"

Adolescent: "I don't really exercise with friends."

Clinician: "In what kind of exercise do you participate?"

Adolescent: "I run."

Clinician: "Do you run by yourself or with a group?"

Adolescent: "By myself."

Clinician: "When do you run?"

Adolescent: "Usually after school."

Clinician: "How far do you run?"

Adolescent: "I don't know, maybe 5 miles?"

Clinician: "How long does that usually take you?"

Adolescent: "45 minutes."

Clinician: "How many times a week do you do that?"

Adolescent: "4 to 5 days per week."

Clinician: "So, what type of exercise would you do when you don't run?"

Adolescent: "I usually do the 'treadmill' for about 15 to 20 minutes."

Clinician: "How often?"

Adolescent: "On the days I don't run outside."

Clinician: "How many times a day would you run on the treadmill?"

Adolescent: "Once . . . ."

Clinician: "What speed and elevation?"

Adolescent: "About 6 mph and no elevation."

Clinician: "Do you do any other form of exercise?"

Adolescent: "Not really."

Clinician: "Do you ever do exercise before you go to bed?"

Adolescent: "May be a few sit-ups."

Clinician: "How many?"

Adolescent: "50."

Clinician: "How many sets of "50" would you do before you go to bed?"

Adolescent: "Four of five . . .."

Adolescents with eating disorders often engage in solitary exercise. The exercise is commonly repetitive, rigid, and unpleasant. The sole point of the exercise is to burn calories and fat. Often adolescents will carefully count the calories they eat and organize an exercise regimen that allows them to burn the calories consumed. It is important to ask about changes in exercise regimen; as weight loss continues, the activity level often increases.

Binging

Adolescents who "binge" will eat a large amount of food in a short period of time and feel a loss of control over their eating.[1,12,13] Some adolescents only binge, whereas others will binge eat and then purge (self-induce vomiting, use laxatives, diuretics, enemas, or diet pills, fast, or exercise). Adolescents do not like to talk about binge eating, because it can leave a young person feeling particularly ashamed and guilty. It may be helpful to preface questions about binging by explaining that it is often a common response to starvation:

Clinician: "Now I would like to ask you about binge eating. We know from research that the body and mind's response to dieting may be to cause a person to eat a large amount of food in a short period of time. Often, adolescents who eat a large amount of food in a short period of time will feel out of control in this situation. We call this a 'binge.' Have you ever experienced anything like this?"

Adolescent: "Well, maybe . . ."

Clinician: "Tell me about this episode? When did you first experience an episode like this?"

Adolescent: "A few months ago . . . maybe 6 months ago."

> Clinician: "This must be upsetting, but again, it is your body trying to get some nutrition and energy."

This is an opportune time to characterize the frequency, time of day, and feelings before, during, and after binge eating. It is also helpful to have her describe a typical binge.

> Clinician: "Most of the adolescents I see feel embarrassed describing the size and nature of their binges. I see binge eating as your body and mind's natural response to feeling starved, so you do not need to feel bad about telling me what you eat. When was the last time you had a binge?"
>
> Adolescent: "Um, 2 days ago."
>
> Clinician: "What time of day did this happen?"
>
> Adolescent: "After school, when no one was home."
>
> Clinician: "Is that when you usually binge?"
>
> Adolescent. "Yes, either after school or at night when my parents and brother are asleep. I wouldn't do this when anyone was around!"
>
> Clinician: "Is this usually the first time you've eaten anything that day?"
>
> Adolescent: "Usually. I always tell myself I'll just have a little cereal, but then I can't stop and I ruin my plan."
>
> Clinician: "So, help me understand this. Can you describe what you're eating in a bit more detail? For instance, how many bowls of cereal did you eat?"
>
> Adolescent: "About 5 bowls."
>
> Clinician: "With milk?"
>
> Adolescent: "At first, then I just eat it straight from the box."
>
> Clinician: "How much cereal do you eat from the box?"
>
> Adolescent: "The whole thing!"
>
> Clinician: "Okay, and then you mentioned cookies. What kind and how many?"

Adolescent: "Whatever we have at home, usually chocolate chip. I eat a lot."

Clinician: "How much is 'a lot?' "

Adolescent: "Usually the whole bag."

Clinician: "And then bread?"

Adolescent: "Yes, I make toast with margarine."

Clinician: "How many slices?"

Adolescent: "Most of the loaf . . . . I don't remember, and I don't like talking about this."

Clinician: "I know that this can be difficult and embarrassing to talk about, but it is important for me to understand the difficulties you are having with eating. Do you worry that you lose control over how much you eat?"

Adolescent: "Yes, totally. It is disgusting and embarrassing!"

Clinician: "Can you identify anything that 'sets you off' or causes you to binge? We call this a trigger. For instance, some young people will binge eat if they feel stressed, upset, hurt, angry, or hungry? Do you have any triggers?"

Adolescent: "It always happens when I am starving. Usually, I haven't eaten all day."

Clinician: "And how do you feel right after you have binged?"

Adolescent: "I feel disgusting, I am so embarrassed! Oh yeah, often my stomach hurts after binging."

As demonstrated, the clinician often has to continually clarify what the adolescent means when she is describing her eating attitudes and behaviors. If done in a calm, nonjudgmental manner, the adolescent will usually give a clear picture of the binging behavior. This data gathering will help clarify whether the adolescent is experiencing "true" or objective binging (as defined by the *Diagnostic and Statistical Manual of Mental Disorders, Fourth Edition* [DSM-IV] criteria [Table 2]) or subjective binging (eating an amount the adolescent feels is too much but does not actually classify as a binge).

Self-induced Vomiting

Purging behaviors are used by adolescents in an attempt to limit calorie absorption. One of the most common methods of purging is self-induced vomiting. The frequency of vomiting varies from adolescent to adolescent, with some vomiting once or twice per week and others many times a day. Self-induced vomiting does not always occur after a binge. Common methods used to provoke vomiting include stimulation of the gag reflex with a finger(s), piece of cutlery, or toothbrush, ingestion of large quantities of fluid, drinking ipecac, or use of abdominal compression. Inquire about self-induced vomiting with questions such as, "Do you make yourself 'sick' (vomit)? How do you make yourself vomit? How often does this occur? What are the triggers? What is the longest period of time you have ever gone between episodes of vomiting? How do you feel before, during, and after this episode?" It is important to explore whether the patient is vomiting blood, which can be the result of tears in the gastric mucosa resulting in Mallory-Weiss syndrome.[12]

Medication and Substance Use

Adolescents with eating disorders may use a variety of medications and/or substances in an attempt to influence their weight. It is important to specifically ask about the type, number taken, last use, frequency of use, and duration of use of laxatives, diuretics, diet pills, enemas, ipecac, and insulin. Adolescents with eating disorders may use nutritional supplements or complementary and alternative medicines that they believe will help them to lose weight or improve their mood.[14] The clinician should also ask about cigarette smoking and illegal drug and alcohol use.

ATTITUDES AND BELIEFS ABOUT WEIGHT AND SHAPE

The DSM-IV diagnostic criteria for anorexia nervosa, bulimia nervosa, and eating disorders, not otherwise specified, include a criterion for "body image disturbance, fear of weight gain, and self-evaluation being unduly influenced by body size and shape" (Tables 1–3).[1] Questions about self-perception and body image can be emotionally charged for an adolescent who feels sad, chronically hungry, ashamed, or angry. This portion of the interview may bring up feelings that the adolescent has been trying to keep hidden from others and even from herself. Allow her the chance to express her feelings, and try not to rush through the silent or emotionally charged moments.

Start with open-ended questions about body image such as, "How would you describe your body size? Is there anything about your body that you would like to change? Why?" For those adolescents who need more direct questioning, one could ask, "Do you feel like you are too thin, too big, or just right?" Other questions to add are, "Has anyone ever told you that you are at a dangerously low weight? If yes, what were your thoughts? How did you feel about that?"

Fear of weight gain may be elicited with, "If I told you that you needed to gain weight to be healthy, how would that make you feel? Are you afraid that if you were to eat normally that you'd gain weight/become fat? How often do you weigh yourself?" Adolescents with eating disorders may weigh themselves daily or multiple times per day.

Often, the adolescent with a restrictive eating disorder is quite aware that others think she is too thin. The adolescent might verbally concur with this assessment even if she does not agree. She may be confused by her feelings about her body and not feel she can discuss them. The adolescent may think the clinician will "get off her back" if she agrees that she is too thin. Finally, the adolescent may hope the clinician will decide her problem is the result of an organic disease rather than an eating disorder if she agrees that she is too thin. It is usually best not to push too hard during this initial interview and risk compromising rapport with the adolescent. Her feelings and concerns will become apparent with time.

Questions about self-evaluation can be difficult for the adolescent to understand, particularly if she is young and a concrete thinker. The following dialogue highlights this.

> Clinician: "How important is your body size to how you feel about yourself as a person?"
>
> Adolescent: "Totally important...."
>
> Clinician: "Do you spend a lot of time thinking about your body?"
>
> Adolescent: "Yes, pretty much all day."
>
> Clinician: "Do you find that you spend a lot of time looking at your body?"
>
> Adolescent: "Yes, all the time!"
>
> Clinician: "How do you examine your body?"
>
> Adolescent: "I weigh myself a few times a day, and I am constantly looking in the mirror."
>
> Clinician: "When you look in the mirror, what do you see?"

Adolescent: "Most of the time, I see a very fat person!"

Clinician: "How does that make you feel?"

Adolescent: "Ugly, disgusting, and lazy! When I feel like this, I won't go to school or out with my friends."

Clinician: "Are there things that you avoid because of the way you feel about your body?"

Adolescent: "Lately, I haven't been doing much of anything except my exercise."

With this type of sequential questioning, the clinician has been able to elicit that the adolescent's self-evaluation is intimately linked with her body image.

MEDICAL HISTORY

As with all adolescent health assessments, it is important to review the past medical history. It is the clinician's role to rule out other potential causes of weight loss, amenorrhea, vomiting, or abnormal eating behaviors. Furthermore, the clinician should also be prepared to identify any medical complications associated with the eating disorder,[15] which will determine the need for additional medical treatment and hospitalization.

MENSTRUAL HISTORY

An accurate menstrual history is of particular importance in the care of an adolescent with an eating disorder. Determine age of menarche, frequency, duration, regularity of menses, amount of blood flow, and last normal menstrual period. If the adolescent has secondary amenorrhea, it would be important to know for how long she has been without a menstrual period. It is essential to inquire about a current or past history of contraceptive use (type and duration). A thorough sexual history including sexual, physical, and emotional abuse should be explored with all adolescents.[16]

PERSONAL PSYCHIATRIC HISTORY AND TREATMENTS

Adolescents with eating disorders commonly have poor self-esteem, withdraw from friends and family, and tend to be inflexible, rigid, and irritable. Approximately 50% to 60% of young people with an eating disorder have a comorbid psychiatric disorder, most commonly depression or anxiety.[17] Furthermore, the mood disturbances often associated with weight loss and malnutrition can be confused with primary depression or anxiety. It is important, therefore, to determine if the adolescent has an eating disorder, a psychiatric disorder other than an eating disorder, or an eating disorder with a comorbid psychiatric disorder. Diagnosis is important, because concurrent treatment of the eating disorder and another psychiatric disorder will increase the likelihood of a full recovery. The clinician should explore the possibility of a mood, anxiety, and substance use/abuse disorder.[18] The clinician should ask the adolescent about any previous diagnosis of an eating or psychiatric disorder and if and how the eating disorder was treated.

Finally, it is important to ask the adolescent about self-harm, suicidality, and homicidal ideation. The clinician needs to inquire about whether the adolescent has a history of these behaviors or whether the adolescent has current suicidal ideation. Self-harm behavior is not uncommon among adolescents with eating disorders.[19] In addition, almost half of the mortality associated with patients with eating disorders relates to suicide. Active plans for suicide should be taken seriously.[20]

FAMILY HISTORY

The clinician should ask the adolescent if she is aware of any family members with medical or psychiatric disorders and what type of treatment was implemented. Questions to ask regarding her family history include, "Do you know of anyone or worry that someone in your family has or has had an eating disorder? Is there anyone in your family with a medical illness? Is there any family member with a history of depression, anxiety, obsessive-compulsive disorder, or suicide? Were they treated? How were they treated?"[21]

REVIEW OF SYSTEMS

Eating disorders are associated with many medical symptoms and complications. A thorough review of systems will often identify several symptoms, even in an adolescent who has only been ill for a short while. Table 6 lists common signs and symptoms that are associated with eating disorders.

INTERVIEWING THE PARENT(S)/GUARDIAN(S) AND OTHER SUPPLEMENTARY INFORMATION

Interviewing the parent(s)/guardian(s) is important, because it provides a clear message that you value the adults in the adolescent's life and they are important to the treatment of the adolescent with an eating disorder.[5] In addition, understanding the adolescent's family constellation (blended, step-, adoptive, and foster families) and culture and ethnic background is important for helping understand the adolescent and her family. Although most parent(s)/guardian(s) have a good understanding of the problem, some may not recognize or acknowledge that their daughter has an eating disorder. Instead, they may focus on the fact that the adolescent has not had a menstrual period for some time, is complaining of being dizzy and cold, has become

Table 6
Physical symptoms associated with eating disorders

System	Anorexia Nervosa/Food Restriction	Bulimia Nervosa/Binge-Purge Cycles
General	Weight loss; feeling cold; irritability/mood changes; depression	Weight fluctuations; irritability/mood changes
Head, eyes, ears, nose, and throat	Dry, cracked lips and tongue; bad breath	Dry lips and tongue; painful teeth and gums; parotid gland tenderness and swelling
Cardiovascular	Dizziness; chest pain; palpitations; cold and/or blue hands and feet; ankle swelling	Dizziness; chest pain; palpitations; ankle swelling
Gastrointestinal	Early satiety; episodes of abdominal pain and discomfort; constipation; bloating after meals	Heart burn; diarrhea or constipation
Endocrine	Absent or irregular menses; fractures	Absent or irregular menses
Dermatologic	Dry skin; brittle nails; yellow-or orange discoloration of skin; thin, dry hair; Extra fine downy hair growth (lanugo); blue discoloration of hands and feet when exposed to cold	
Musculoskeletal	Fatigue, muscle weakness, and cramps	Fatigue, muscle weakness, and cramps
Neurologic	Decreased concentration, memory, thinking ability	Decreased concentration, memory, thinking ability

withdrawn, or has symptoms of anxiety. So, before the clinician presumes that he or she has a similar understanding of the situation as the parent(s)/guardian(s), it is important to ask a few questions: "When did you first notice any changes with your daughter? Did you notice any difficulty with her eating? If yes, when? When did she first begin to lose weight? What did you notice? What did you do at that time? Was it helpful? Why or why not? Describe mealtime before your daughter became sick? Describe meal time now? Does it feel that your daughter's eating attitudes or behaviors have come to occupy a central place in your family's life? How is the rest of the family coping with your daughter's eating? Is there a lot of stress or fighting? Have the relationships between your daughter and her siblings been adversely affected by the eating disorder? Do you feel guilty or worry that you are to blame for your daughter's eating disorder?" It is helpful to confirm the 24-hour dietary recall with the adolescent's parent(s)/guardian(s). They may give a more accurate estimation of food variety and portion size than the adolescent. Conversely, they may tell you their daughter never eats in front of them (quite common), and this is a crucial behavior to address in treatment.

Like the adolescent, parent(s)/guardian(s) may be worried about the stigma that may come with an eating-disorder diagnosis. The parent(s)/guardian(s) may feel that they somehow caused their daughter's eating disorder. It is not uncommon for parent(s)/

guardian(s) to express guilt about their daughter's physical and mental state. It is the clinician's responsibility to educate the parent(s)/guardian(s) that there is no evidence that parent(s)/guardian(s) cause a child's eating disorder.

In most cases, the adolescent and parents(s)/guardian(s) will provide sufficient medical and mental health information. However, keep in mind that it may be important to seek collateral information from the adolescent's school or other agencies with which the adolescent and her family have been involved, including any relevant psychological or school reports and results.

CONCLUSION OF THE INTERVIEW

At the completion of the interview with the adolescent, the clinician should ask the adolescent whether she has any questions or has any additional information that will help the clinician understand what is currently going on. The clinician should inform the adolescent and family that a physical examination and laboratory investigations are also part of the full assessment for an eating disorder. When all components of the assessment are complete, the clinician will be able to provide a diagnosis and a more comprehensive treatment plan (which may include a referral to a specialized child and adolescent eating-disorder program) to the adolescent and her family.

Advances in our understanding and treatment of adolescent eating disorders have resulted in improvements in the way clinicians approach the assessment. Interviewing an adolescent with a suspected eating disorder is a process designed to help the adolescent through a very difficult time. The assessment of an adolescent with an eating disorder is the first step toward recovery.

REFERENCES

1. American Psychiatric Association. *Diagnostic and Statistical Manual of Mental Disorders*. 4th ed. Washington, DC: American Psychiatric Association; 1994
2. American Academy of Pediatrics, Committee on Adolescence. Identifying and treating eating disorders. *Pediatrics.* 2003;111(1):204–211
3. Golden NH, Katzman DK, Kreipe RE, et al. Eating disorders in adolescents: position paper of the Society for Adolescent Medicine. *J Adolesc Health.* 2003;33(6):496–503
4. Nicholls D, Chater R, Lask B. Children into DSM don't go: a comparison of classification systems for eating disorders in childhood and early adolescence. *Int J Eat Disord.* 2000;28(3):317–324
5. Pinhas L, Morris A, Heinmaa M, Crosby R, Katzman DK. Early onset eating disorders. Presented at: Canadian Paediatric Society 83rd Annual Conference; June 13–17, 2006; St John's, Newfoundland
6. Le Grange D, Lock J, Dymek M. Family-based therapy for adolescents with bulimia nervosa. *Am J Psychother.* 2003;57(2):237–251
7. Klostermann BK, Slap GB, Nebrig DM. Earning trust and losing it: adolescents' views on trusting physicians. *J Fam Pract.* 2005;54(8):679–687
8. Neinstein LS, ed. *Adolescent Health Care: A Practical Guide.* 4th ed. Philadelphia, PA: Lippincott, Williams & Wilkins; 2002

9. Neumark-Sztainer D, Story M, Hannan PJ, Beuhring T, Resnick MD. Disordered eating among adolescents: associations with sexual/physical abuse and other familial/psychosocial factors. *Int J Eat Disord.* 2000;28(3):249–258
10. Golden NH, Jacobson MS, Schebendach J, Solanto MV, Hertz SM, Shenker IR. Resumption of menses in anorexia nervosa. *Arch Pediatr Adolesc Med.* 1997;151(1):16–21
11. Neumark-Sztainer D, Story M, Resnick MD, Blum RW. Adolescent vegetarians: a behavioral profile of a school-based population in Minnesota. *Arch Pediatr Adolesc Med.* 1997;151(8):833–838
12. Schneider M. Bulimia nervosa and binge-eating disorder in adolescents. *Adolesc Med.* 2003;14(1):119–131
13. Marcus MD, Kalarchian MA. Binge eating in children and adolescents. *Int J Eat Disord.* 2003;34(suppl):S47–S57
14. Trigazis L, Tennankore D, Vohra S, Katzman DK. The use of herbal remedies by adolescents with eating disorders. *Int J Eat Disord.* 2004;35(2):223–228
15. Katzman DK. Medical complications in adolescents with anorexia nervosa: a review of the literature. *Int J Eat Disord.* 2005;37(suppl):S52–S59; discussion S87–S89
16. Wonderlich SA, Crosby RD, Mitchell JE, et al. Eating disturbance and sexual trauma in childhood and adulthood. *Int J Eat Disord.* 2001;30(4):401–412
17. Steinhausen HC. The outcome of anorexia nervosa in the 20th century. *Am J Psychiatry.* 2002;159(8):1284–1293
18. Stock SL, Goldberg E, Corbett S, Katzman DK. Substance use in female adolescents with eating disorders. *J Adolesc Health.* 2002;31(2):176–182
19. Ruuska J, Kaltiala-Heino R, Rantanen P, Koivisto AM. Psychopathological distress predicts suicidal ideation and self-harm in adolescent eating disorder outpatients. *Eur Child Adolesc Psychiatry.* 2005;14(5):276–281
20. Herzog DB, Greenwood DN, Dorer DJ, et al. Mortality in eating disorders: a descriptive study. *Int J Eat Disord.* 2000;28(1):20–26
21. Sullivan PF, Bulik CM, Carter FA, Gendall KA, Joyce PR. The significance of a prior history of anorexia in bulimia nervosa. *Int J Eat Disord.* 1996;20(3):253–261

Talking With Adolescents and Their Families About Emotional and Behavioral Concerns

Rheanna Platt, MD, MPH[a], Kate Fothergill, PhD[b], Lawrence S. Wissow, MD, MPH[b,c]

[a]*Department of Pediatrics, Johns Hopkins School of Medicine, 600 N. Wolfe Street, Baltimore, MD 21287, USA*

[b]*Department of Health, Behavior, and Society, Johns Hopkins Bloomberg School of Public Health, 624 N. Broadway, Baltimore, MD 21205, USA*

[c]*Berman Bioethics Institute, Johns Hopkins University, 624 N. Broadway, Baltimore, MD 21205, USA*

Up to a quarter of US adolescents are thought to have mental health problems,[1] a proportion that seems to be increasing.[2] Only a minority of affected adolescents (~30%) reportedly receive treatment.[3] Many who are treated do so in the context of primary care.[4] Many sources have provided guidelines for the content of mental health–centered primary care visits, such as the American Medical Association's *Guidelines for Adolescent Preventive Services* and the mental health practice guide and toolkit from *Bright Futures in Practice*,[5,6] but few sources have provided guidance on how to talk with adolescents about mental health. In this article we address 4 challenges that are commonly encountered by primary care physicians who treat adolescents: (1) working with/responding to adolescents' potentially limited or biased knowledge of mental health problems and their treatment; (2) balancing adolescents' desire for confidentiality with families' interest in being involved in the adolescents' care; (3) managing encounters with families and adolescents together, especially when the adolescent is a reluctant participant; and (4) working with families who are discouraged or feel hopeless.

ADOLESCENTS' KNOWLEDGE OF MENTAL HEALTH AND ITS TREATMENT

Surveys have revealed that many adolescents have a limited understanding of what constitutes a treatable mental health problem.[7,8] Periods of low mood, low energy, and lack of interest in life are often seen as normative and, as such,

---

*Corresponding author.
E-mail address: lwissow@jhsph.edu (L. Wissow).

something that one should manage alone or with the help of friends and family. To many adolescents, in contrast, the label "mental health problem" is synonymous with severe developmental delay or psychotic thinking (ie, referring to people as "retarded" or "crazy"). Thus, although counseling and psychopharmacologic medication may be acceptable or even fashionable to some adolescents, formal treatment accompanied by a psychiatric diagnosis is often seen as highly stigmatized and a sign of failure or being defective.[9]

Given these high stakes, it is perhaps not surprising that one of adolescents' prime concerns about divulging emotional concerns to their doctor centers on the doctor's abilities. Adolescents who seek medical care voice concern that doctors demonstrate competence,[10] and they seem to have similar attitudes about receipt of mental health care. In the process of creating materials for training pediatric primary care providers to talk more effectively with families about mental health, we conducted brief interviews with 12 adolescents about their primary care doctors and mental health (this pilot work for what became the Bassett/Hopkins Program in Mental Health Communication Skills for Child and Adolescent Primary Care was approved by the Johns Hopkins Bloomberg School of Public Health Committee on Human Research). The interviews took place at 2 community-based multispecialty primary care offices, 1 in a low- to middle-income city neighborhood and 1 in a blue-collar and middle-class suburban area. Provider competence was among the most commonly cited factors related to comfort disclosing emotional distress. These adolescents looked for signs that their doctor was knowledgeable about mental health, including the doctor raising the topic, disclosing similar experiences in his or her own adolescence, or mentioning having teenaged children of his or her own. They also assessed competence by interactional style. They wanted doctors who "sounded knowledgeable" and who were capable of providing clear explanations that were mature but free of jargon. As one adolescent said, "[I want them to talk to me] in any way so they wouldn't be up there in the scientific mode and I'm down here, like, what are you talking about?" Similar to findings by others,[11] these adolescents were also concerned about their doctors' professionalism. The concerns included wanting to feel confident that the doctor would not be disclosing the adolescent's story to other staff members. As one said, "I would be more comfortable telling them if I knew that they wouldn't be going around like telling the other doctors, laughing . . .."

The concerns outlined above suggest the use of several communication techniques to establish an atmosphere of respect and to show receptivity, competence, and a willingness to frame the discussion in terms that are comfortable for the adolescent. Some of these techniques may seem self-evident and a part of everyday practice, but research suggests that they may go unused in the course of rapid encounters.[12]

1. Set up the environment for disclosure by showing interest, making good eye contact (especially if using an electronic chart), and closing the door.

Despite being busy, cultivate a manner that implies having the time to listen.
2. Start with an open-ended greeting such as "How have things been since the last time?" or "How can I be of help?" rather than, "So I see we are here for your annual physical."
3. Try not to interrupt the adolescent's initial answer by asking specific questions or giving information. Show either nonverbally, or by briefly summarizing what has been said so far, that any concern is open for discussion.
4. Follow-up on hints about undisclosed problems. Hints may take the form of changes in voice tone or facial expression or seemingly incidental comments about life events. Be curious. Although asking may seem to take time, it can prove to be efficient if serious emotional problems surface later in the visit or prove to be what underlies a difficult-to-diagnose somatic concern.
5. Ask specifically about emotional concerns in domains that are of interest to adolescents, including academics, sports, and relationships with parents, friends, and boyfriends or girlfriends.
6. Before starting to make a diagnosis and offering advice, take the time to understand how the adolescent defines his or her emotional or behavioral problem. Later, you will have an opportunity to map the problem onto your own set of diagnoses, but first you can demonstrate your ability to help by making sure that (*a*) you and the adolescent can agree on a plain-language statement of the problem, (*b*) you have a clear understanding of what the adolescent sees as the causes and solutions, if any, (*c*) you've had a chance to show your familiarity with mental health concerns, and (*d*) you have a feel for whether the adolescent is seeking a solution now or is only willing to speak about the possibility of seeking one in the future.

CONFIDENTIALITY

Concern about confidentiality poses one of the biggest barriers to adolescents' discussion of mental health problems with primary care providers. Assurance of confidentiality increases teens' willingness to seek care for sensitive emotional medical problems, whereas concerns about parental notification have an opposite effect.[10,13–15] In a statewide survey of Massachusetts high school students, 75% said there were some health concerns for which they would want to be able to seek care without their parents' knowledge, but only 28% said their health care provider had ever talked to them about confidentiality.[16] Some teens find that their doctors do not discuss confidentiality at all, whereas other doctors promise unconditional confidentiality that ultimately cannot be honored.[17] Some adolescents may be surprised that the subject ever comes up.

Adolescents' social context and evolving data about the influence of parent-child collaboration pose dilemmas for how clinicians approach confidentiality and teen mental health concerns. Despite their well-documented desire for confidentiality, adolescents often cite family members as their primary source of help for emotional problems.[18] In addition, families often play an essential role in mental health diagnosis and treatment. Parents and children frequently provide different ratings when asked to report on children's behavior, emotional health, and experiences.[19,20] As a rule, parents are more likely than children to report behavior problems and to consider them to be more severe. On the other hand, parents tend to underestimate the frequency and severity of low mood and anxiety, as well as the extent to which their children have been exposed to traumatic events.[21] Discrepancies tend to be greater among families in which children have been referred for mental health problems than among community samples.[22] Adolescents' treatment options may be limited when their families are not involved. Adolescents may have no independent means of paying for laboratory tests, medications, or transportation to and from care. In addition, optimal treatment for adults and children often requires the collaboration of family members to provide support, monitor progress, or take an active role in the intervention. For other chronic illnesses in adolescence, such as diabetes, collaboration between teens and parents is related to better outcomes compared with teens being asked to take on management responsibilities alone.[23,24]

Some family environments, however, directly or indirectly contribute to young people's mental health problems.[25,26] In many of these families, disclosure of an adolescent's emotional distress may engender anger and disorganization rather than support. This may particularly be the case for families in which a parent has a mental health or substance abuse problem of his or her own. In some families, parents have strong religious or cultural beliefs that limit treatment choices open to their children,[27] whereas others may block a child's help-seeking for fear of disclosure of sensitive family information. Families in which parents have untreated or partially treated mental health problems actually may be less, rather than more, willing to seek treatment should their children show signs of distress.[28]

There are several considerations that providers can use for developing a strategy for balancing adolescents' needs and desires for confidential visits (as well as, in most jurisdictions, their legal rights) with the potential benefits of involving other family members at some stage in diagnosis and treatment.

1. Previous discussions and understanding regarding confidentiality: Although teens may be aware that some things cannot be kept confidential (such as suicidality and child abuse), they may not be aware of topics that can potentially be discussed confidentially under local law.[29] Ideally, before the onset of any emotional or behavioral problems, the family, adolescent, and provider can agree on mutually acceptable ways in which the adolescent can disclose concerns and how the provider might proceed in terms of informing the family. For example, at an annual visit in early adolescence, the provider might raise the issue of future emotional distress,

let it be known that he or she could be of help, and ask the family how they would want to proceed should the need arise.
2. Developing a picture of family context: On the basis of the adolescent's report or previous knowledge, assess key areas of family functioning that are important for supporting adolescent development.[25] Areas include (*a*) warmth and empathy (versus negativity and lack of support), (*b*) cohesiveness in the face of crisis and loss, and (*c*) ability to balance closeness with respect for privacy. Has the adolescent advanced any reason to believe that involving the family would put him or her at some form of risk? There are several lines of questions that might help in this assessment. First and foremost are questions about family violence, which are part of general psychosocial screening. Second, the provider might ask the adolescent if there has been a time in the past when he or she had to tell their parents some "bad news," for example, such as receiving a failing grade or having gotten into trouble outside the home. How was this handled by the parents? Did the adolescent ultimately feel supported to improve, or was there a prolonged period of tension? A similar question could be asked about how the family reacted to a major loss such as the death of a grandparent or to a major illness among one of the family members. Was the family able to maintain its routines and mutual caring, or were there conflicts over how to respond or discussions of blame? Finally, if one of the family members has had some difficulty with his or her health, work, or school, has this problem been managed sensitively within the home? Was it possible to keep knowledge of the details among only those family members who truly needed to know them, or was there a sense that details were disclosed indiscriminately?
3. Resources and informational needs: Clinicians and adolescents need to weigh together whether adequate care can be provided confidentially, and, if not, what other avenues might be open. Similarly, clinicians might ask themselves whether they feel that information from the adolescent alone (or from the adolescent plus nonfamily sources such as peers or teachers) is sufficient to develop an accurate diagnosis and corresponding treatment plan. Some specific issues might include:
    a. Has the adolescent stated directly that involving the parents would preclude his or her accepting any treatment?
    b. Can the diagnosis be made by using only the adolescent's account of his or her personal and family history? In what ways might the diagnosis or initial treatment plan differ if other information were available from parents or other family members?
    c. Can some form of effective treatment be offered within the financial or other logistic limitations imposed by confidentiality or adolescent autonomy?
    d. Is there reason to be concerned that not involving the family from the outset could have negative consequences for the adolescent (eg, there would be opportunity for continuity of care or if an adolescent has a condition that could rapidly deteriorate)? Will the adolescent consider the condition that

the clinician can unilaterally break confidentiality in certain circumstances beyond the usual exceptions (eg, the adolescent dropping out of care at a time when he or she appears to be significantly distressed)?

e. If the family is already involved to some extent (eg, have brought the adolescent for care but are not privy to particular disclosures or treatment decisions), can the adolescent and clinician agree to what honestly can be told to the family now and how the family can be kept abreast of progress in a way that maintains their support for the treatment but protects the adolescent's request for confidentiality/autonomy? If the family is not now involved, can the adolescent and clinician agree on how the clinician should respond to questions should he or she be contacted by the family? Would it be reasonable for the provider to let the family know that he or she will be having ongoing contact with the adolescent without divulging the nature of the problem or treatment?

4. The adolescent's decision-making capacity: Clinicians have a responsibility to create settings in which the adolescent has an opportunity to make thoughtful decisions, including providing information in age-appropriate language, allowing sufficient time for decision-making, and possibly providing someone other than the clinician to offer support. In the case of confidential mental health care, a particular issue is whether the teen is able to thoughtfully discuss the pros and cons of not involving his or her family. The level of "capacity" required is proportional to the risks involved—risks relating to the teen's condition and risks relating to concerns about the family's response. Some questions to ask here might include:

a. Is there any a priori reason for concern about diminished capacity (eg, teen is intoxicated, in a state of crisis, or seems focused entirely on present as opposed to longer-term consequences, has serious cognitive or language issues, or is involved in criminal or antisocial behavior)? Is this a situation (eg, suicidality, homicidality, child abuse) in which involvement of others is mandatory?

b. Are basic criteria for decision-making capacity met (the teen seems to have a reasonable set of values by which to judge options, can take in information and express his or her views, and has the ability to reason about possible choices)?[30]

   i. Has the adolescent been able to express in a clear and balanced way his or her reasoning about involvement of other family members?
   ii. Can the adolescent be engaged in a discussion of the practical pros and cons of seeking care within versus outside the context of the family?

MANAGING ENCOUNTERS WITH BOTH PARENTS AND ADOLESCENTS

Parents or other adult family members are often the ones to raise concerns about an adolescent's emotions or behavior. Adolescents are often passive or unwilling partners in this process. Even if they have agreed to come to the doctor's office, they may decline to participate. The subsequent discussion then becomes 1-sided, which often results in a negatively tinged conversation between the adult and the doctor talking about the adolescent as if he or she were not present. Alternatively, the adult and adolescent may interrupt each other, trade negative remarks about each other, and try to recruit the doctor to their side. In this section, we discuss techniques designed to help avoid these situations and manage them when they inevitably occur.

The process of working with an adolescent who feels coerced into the visit can be seen as having 3 stages: acknowledging anger, distancing oneself tactfully from the coercive referral, and offering choice.[31(p129)] One goal is to start a process through which the adolescent can start to feel a sense of control, and you can come to be seen as someone who can be trusted to thoughtfully weigh what is being said without jumping to conclusions. Another goal is to test the possibility of establishing a respectful 3-way dialogue, because whatever treatment you propose is likely to involve parent-adolescent collaboration. In addition, younger teens may feel more comfortable with their parent present, and families from some cultures may be reluctant to have you see their child alone. None of this precludes ultimately talking separately with the adolescent and parent. Some possible "openers" to an angry adolescent include:

> "I realize that it wasn't your idea to come here, but I am really interested in hearing how you feel about this issue."
>
> "I guess it is doubly hard getting told you have to talk to someone and then not even having the choice of who that is. Do you think you might feel more comfortable with someone else? I can help you set that up if you would like."
>
> "I hear your father's agenda for the visit today, but is there anything that you would like to accomplish, on this topic or on any other?"

Sometimes adolescents who feel coerced will simply refuse to speak, or they may make a statement about why they feel their parents' concerns are ill-founded. Both of these can be seen as a form of "resistance" in psychotherapy parlance—an unwillingness to engage in the treatment being proposed. Resistance can develop as a defense against shame, in response to feeling cornered, or out of pride—the feeling that this is something the adolescent could or should be able to handle on his or her own. Clinicians often meet resistance head on by pushing harder and insisting on participation. An alternative is to "roll" with the resistance by treating it as an ordinary occurrence to be met instead with flexibility and empathy.[32] This can be done in several ways:

1. One way is to simply repeat or reflect the adolescent's thought, if one is expressed: "So you don't agree with your mother that you've been irritable

lately?" The hope is that the adolescent will elaborate, giving some detail about his or her feelings and giving you an opportunity to show respect for his or her position and ask questions that clarify it.
2. You can apologize and back up a bit: "I'm sorry. This probably isn't the best way to start off our visit. What else did we need to get done today? Is it okay with you if we start there and come back to this?"
3. You can agree "with a twist." "Yes, I hear you, you really have been feeling fine. So what do you think your mother has been noticing?"
4. You can ask for permission to clarify a few potentially urgent matters such as suicidal thoughts or recent trauma. "I respect your not wanting to talk at all about this, but given your mother's concerns, may I ask you just a couple of questions that I would ask anyone about their safety? Then whether we go on is up to you."

Parent-adolescent arguments during a visit can derail plans for diagnosis and treatment, and they frequently leave everyone involved feeling impotent and discouraged. Sometimes they can be avoided by taking steps at the outset of the visit to ensure that both parties get a chance to speak and by making sure that there has been adequate discussion about whether they should be interviewed separately or together.

When the parent and adolescent choose to remain together for the visit, clinicians can suggest and enforce turn-taking by shifting their gaze and body position from parent to adolescent and back, demonstrating attention to both and the expectation that both will speak. If the parent interrupts the adolescent or vice versa, their concern can be recognized, and they can be asked to wait briefly while the other finishes.

One way to break up arguments is to interrupt them and point out areas of agreement: "I hear you both saying that relationships in the family are important, but you, [teen], are concerned about being respected by your parents, and you, [parent], are concerned about how much time he spends at home. Do you think there is a common thread to those things that we could talk about?" Arguments can also be normalized to try to take some of the emotion out of them. "It's pretty common for parents and children to disagree about curfews and calling to say where you are. It's part of the whole process of learning how to be independent and responsible. How has your family been handling that?"

If one or both parties seem particularly angry or are saying things that seem hurtful, there are several ways to appeal for a calmer approach. One technique is to suggest that the argument is happening in the context of a caring relationship:

> "This must be hard. It's difficult when two people care a lot about each other but really disagree. Is there a way you could tell [teen] how you feel but also let him know how much you care about him?"

Another technique is to point out the use of polarizing or "black-and-white" words and thinking. These tend to promote escalating insults, and they also obscure concerns that could be the focus of a plan. Examples include: "He is always late/he never picks up after himself." "He is lazy/he doesn't care about anyone else in the family." Responses on your part can be:

> "Ever, never, always—those words have a way of putting people on the defensive. Can you try telling her those concerns again, but without using those words?"[33(p35)]

> "People often get upset if they feel you are labeling them, and it can really stick with kids even if they tell you they don't care. Can you tell him what he does that upsets you without using that label to explain why he does it?"

HELPING ADOLESCENTS (AND THEIR FAMILIES) WHO SAY THEY ARE "STUCK," FEEL HOPELESS, OR HAVE "TRIED EVERYTHING"

Anger, low mood, and anxiety cause a "tunnel vision" that makes it hard to see a way out of problems; hopelessness and demoralization become vicious cycles that continue to deepen. Focusing on goals for the immediate future and how to get there can often be more productive than a detailed analysis of how problems came about; sometimes the goals are all that is needed. "Solution-focused" therapy grew out of a need for ways to help people do this in the course of brief clinical interactions.[34,35]

Solution-focused interventions have 2 components. First, "reframing" is designed to create at least a temporary sense of pride and optimism—seeing the glass as half full instead of half empty. Then, second, goals are developed that are practical, readily measured, and likely to be achieved—the "first step" that starts a longer journey. The adolescent or family is considered to be the expert on both desired goals and ways to get there; the clinician is a facilitator and coach. The family, not the doctor, does the "work" of coming up with solutions to its problems.

Reframing often starts by asking someone to tell the story of his or her problem. "Story" refers to the patient's understanding of how he or she came to be in a particular situation. Although at first many people will say that they do not know, they can be prompted by asking them to describe when the problem started and how it has evolved. "I know that we could probably talk about this for hours, but in a few minutes, starting at the beginning, tell me how you got to this point." Asking for a story may at first seem contradictory to keeping a focus on the present, but the search for solutions will remain, in fact, very much in the present. To change, people need to feel understood and supported. You do not have to agree with everything the family has done, but you can support the difficulty of the situation, the strengths that have been demonstrated, and point out how the problems "make sense" given the circumstances. The first, and often the only, response necessary is your ability to play the story back in a way that provides validation and empathy.

> "So here you are, a single parent trying to hold down two jobs, with a child who is not the easiest in the world to manage. Then, on top of that, your own mother gets sick and needs you. What a tough situation."

> "I can understand why you are so discouraged. It seems as if nothing is going right, and everyone seems to be blaming you."

In listening to the story you can also look for situations that seem important to you but seem to have been glossed over in the patient's or family's account. For example, imagine an adolescent told you about progressive problems with work at school and relationships, and he or she mentioned quickly in the middle of the account that a sibling has a serious, chronic illness. In your playing back of the story, you note this and speculate that it must have had an impact. It is not a problem if the adolescent corrects you or provides more information that changes your interpretation; that is part of the conversation. What matters in this exchange is that the adolescent has had a chance to clarify the story for himself or herself.

Another technique when listening to stories is to observe and comment on "shoulds." "Shoulds" can be stated explicitly, as in "whenever he does x, I have to do y," or as in, "I should have done . . . .." They can also be stated implicitly through a pattern of behavior that recurs in a story[33]: "So you are saying that every time he gets into trouble it is your job to bail him out. That sounds like an important rule that you are following; where did it come from?" Note that in your comment you are not suggesting that the rule is bad, or even suggesting an alternative point of view. But by asking someone if this really is a "rule" that they follow and asking them to comment on its origin, you give them the opportunity and permission to make a modification.

Eliciting stories usually segues into "so, where do we go from here?" or "so, what do you want to have happen next?" You can help families set concrete, observable goals. In general, useful goals have the following characteristics:

- People develop them for themselves.
- They are framed in terms of positive behaviors that are observable. For example, if a parent starts out saying that she would like her teenaged daughter to stop being so negative in her responses to requests, a corresponding goal might be that the daughter will initiate the requested activity within a certain time and with no more than one prompt.

- They are often framed in very small steps: "What is the first change in that direction that you would like to see?"
- They can be counted or documented objectively; thus, progress can be assessed.

When people say they are at a loss for a goal, one can ask them what they feel would be the first, small sign that things were beginning to improve—preferably so small that they feel confident they could achieve it.[35(p134)] For example, if an adolescent is despairing over the inability to lose weight, a first goal could be to walk up the steps from the subway rather than take the escalator. People can also be asked to try to recall exceptions, a time at which the desired outcome or state actually occurred, even if only briefly. The discussion can then move on to what might have been happening then and if those circumstances can be recreated.

CONCLUSIONS

A variety of communication skills and strategies have the potential to increase disclosure of adolescents' psychosocial problems and engage adolescents and their families in the process of seeking solutions and following through with treatment. These skills and strategies can be incorporated into routine visits and promote primary care as a place to access help with adolescent emotional and behavioral problems.

ACKNOWLEDGMENTS

This work was supported by National Institute of Mental Health grants K24 MH 001790 and RO1 MH 62469.

REFERENCES

1. Costello EJ, Mustillo S, Erkanli A, Keeler G, Angold A. Prevalence and development of psychiatric disorders in childhood and adolescence. *Arch Gen Psychiatry.* 2003;60(8):837–844
2. Birmaher B, Neal R, Williamson DE, et al. Childhood and adolescent depression: a review of the past 10 years. Part I. *J Am Acad Child Adolesc Psychiatry.* 1996;35(11):1427–1439
3. Kodjo C, Auinger P, Ryan S. Barriers to adolescents accessing mental health services [abstract]. *J Adolesc Health.* 2002;30:101–102
4. Leaf PJ, Alegria M, Cohen P, et al. Mental health service use in the community and schools: results from the four-community MECA study. *J Am Acad Child Adolesc Psychiatry.* 1996;35(7):889–897
5. American Medical Association. *Guidelines for Adolescent Preventive Services.* Chicago, IL: American Medical Association; 1992
6. Jellinek M, Patel BP, Froehle MC, eds. *Bright Futures in Practice: Mental Health—Volume I, Practice Guide.* Arlington, VA: National Center for Education in Maternal and Child Health; 2002
7. Zachrisson HD, Rödje K, Mykletun A. Utilization of health services in relation to mental health problems in adolescents: a population based survey. *BMC Public Health.* 2006;6:34
8. Verhuslt FC, van der Ende J. Factors associated with child mental health service use in the community. *J Am Acad Child Adolesc Psychiatry.* 1997;36(7):901–909

9. Secker J, Armstrong C, Hill M. Young people's understanding of mental illness. *Health Educ Res*. 1999;14(6):729-739
10. Ginsburg KR, Menapace AS, Slap GB. Factors affecting the decision to seek health care: the voice of adolescents. *Pediatrics*. 1997;100(6):922-930
11. Kapphahn CJ, Wilson KM, Klein JD. Adolescent girls' and boys' preferences for provider gender and confidentiality in their health care. *J Adolesc Health*. 1999;25(2):131-142
12. Wissow LS, Roter D, Larson S, Wang MC, Hwang WT, Johnson R. Mechanisms behind the failure of longitudinal primary care to promote the disclosure and discussion of psychosocial issues. *Arch Pediatr Adolesc Med*. 2002;156(7):685-692
13. Cheng T, Savageau JA, Sattler AL, DeWitt TT. Confidentiality in health care: a survey of knowledge, perceptions, and attitudes among high school students. *JAMA*. 1993;269(11):1404-1407
14. Ford CA, Millstein SG, Halpern-Felsher B, Irwin C. Influence of physician confidentiality assurances on adolescents' willingness to disclose information and seek future health care: a randomized controlled trial. *JAMA*. 1997;278(12):1029-1034
15. Reddy DM, Fleming R, Swain C. Effect of mandatory parental notification on adolescent girls' use of sexual health care services. *JAMA*. 2002;288(6):710-714
16. Thrall JS, McCloskey L, Ettner SL, Rothman E, Tighe JE, Emans J. Confidentiality and adolescents' use of providers for health information and for pelvic examinations. *Arch Pediatr Adolesc Med*. 2000;154(9):885-892
17. Ford C, Millstein SG. Delivery of confidentiality assurances to adolescents by primary care physicians. *Arch Pediatr Adolesc Med*. 1997;151(5):505-509
18. Offer D, Howard K, Schonert K, Ostrov E. To whom do adolescents turn for help? Differences between disturbed and nondisturbed adolescents. *J Am Acad Child Adolesc Psychiatr*. 1991;30:623-630
19. Yeh M, Weisz JR. Why are we here at the clinic? Parent-child (dis)agreement on referral problems at outpatient treatment entry. *J Consult Clin Psychol*. 2001;69(6):1018-1025
20. Brown JD, Wissow LS, Gadomski A, Zachary C, Bartlett E, Horn I. Parent and teacher mental health ratings of children using primary-care services: interrater agreement and implications for mental health screening. *Ambul Pediatr*. 2006;6(6):347-351
21. Richters JE, Martinez P. The NIMH Community Violence Project: I. Children as victims of and witnesses to violence. *Psychiatry*. 1993;56(1):7-21
22. MacLeod RJ, McNamee JE, Boyle MH, Offord DR, Friedrich M. Identification of childhood psychiatric disorder by informant: comparisons of clinic and community samples. *Can J Psychiatry*. 1999;44(2):144-150
23. Fiese BH, Wamboldt FS. Tales of pediatric asthma management: family-based strategies related to medical adherence and health care utilization. *J Pediatr*. 2003;143(4):457-462
24. Hutchinson MK, Jemmott JB 3rd, Jemmott LS, Braverman P, Fong GT. The role of mother-daughter sexual risk communication in reducing sexual risk behaviors among urban adolescent females: a prospective study. *J Adolesc Health*. 2003;33(2):98-107
25. Group for the Advancement of Psychiatry. *Adolescent Suicide*. Washington, DC: American Psychiatric Press, Inc; 1996
26. Repetti RL, Taylor SE, Seeman TE. Risky families: family and social environments and the mental and physical health of offspring. *Psychol Bull*. 2002;128(2):330-366
27. Holder AR. Parents, courts, and refusal of treatment. *J Pediatr*. 1983;103(4):515-521
28. Flisher AJ, Kramer RA, Grosser RC, et al. Correlates of unmet need for mental health services by children and adolescents. *Psychol Med*. 1997;27(5):1145-1154
29. Ford CA, Thomsen SL, Compton B. Adolescents' interpretations of conditional confidentiality assurances. *J Adolesc Health*. 2001;29(3):156-159
30. President's Commission for the Study of Ethical Problems in Medicine and Biomedical and Behavioral Research. *Making Health Care Decisions: A Report on the Ethical and Legal Implications of Informed Consent in the Patient-Practitioner Relationship. Vol. 1: Report*. Washington, DC: Superintendent of Documents; 1982:57

31. Rollnick S, Mason P, Butler C. *Health Behavior Change: A Guide for Practitioners.* Edinburgh, Scotland: Churchill Livingstone; 1999
32. Miller WR, Rollnick S. *Motivational Interviewing: Preparing People to Change Addictive Behavior.* New York, NY: Guilford Press; 1991
33. Allmond BW Jr, Tanner JL, Gofman HF. *The Family Is the Patient: Using Family Interviews in Children's Medical Care.* 2nd ed. Baltimore, MD: Williams & Wilkins; 1999
34. Walter J, Peller J. *Becoming Solution-Focused in Brief Therapy.* New York, NY: Brunner/Mazel; 1992
35. Klar H, Coleman WL. Brief solution-focused strategies for behavioral pediatrics. *Pediatr Clin North Am.* 1995;42(1):131–141

Motivational Interviewing With Adolescents

Patricia K. Kokotailo, MD, MPH[a]*, Melanie A. Gold, DO[b]

[a]*Department of Pediatrics, University of Wisconsin School of Medicine and Public Health, 2870 University Avenue, Suite 200, Madison, WI 53705, USA*

[b]*Division of Adolescent Medicine, Department of Pediatrics, University of Pittsburgh Student Health Service, Medical Arts Building, Suite 500.9, 3708 Fifth Avenue, Pittsburgh, PA 15213, USA*

Physicians and other health care providers who care for adolescents are constantly addressing behavioral issues. Whether counseling about drug or alcohol use, smoking, obesity, eating disorders, or other behaviors, health care providers often struggle with how to best help patients change their behavior. Simply giving advice or educating alone are rarely effective methods for facilitating behavior, especially when there may be ambivalence or resistance to change. Giving advice may often be perceived as lecturing by an adolescent who quickly "tunes out" the provider. An alternative approach to facilitating behavior change is motivational interviewing (MI). MI is a counseling style that initially grew out of the work of psychologist Carl Rogers, who espoused an empathic approach. Miller and Rollnick[1] initially described MI as a novel approach to treating alcohol and other drug abuse. MI is a term that describes a clinical counseling style that is patient centered, directive and enhances intrinsic motivation to change by exploring and resolving ambivalence. It does not focus on teaching new coping skills or reshaping cognitions. The approach focuses on the patient's current interests and concerns and is aimed at developing discrepancies between present behavior and important personal goals and values. MI involves responding to patients in ways that help to resolve ambivalence to behavior change, reduce resistance, and move the patient toward change.

Although described as a brief intervention, formal use of MI usually entails 45- to 60-minute sessions, which may not be feasible in most medical outpatient settings. Briefer adaptations of MI, such as brief advice (5–15 minutes, with a more active expert with a passive recipient) and behavior-change counseling (5–30 minutes, with a counselor with an active participant) may be more readily used in a medical setting. Other terms often used to describe interventions that use motivational strategies include motivational enhancement therapy (MET) and motivational interventions. MET has been defined as MI combined with personal feedback of assessment results.[2]

---

*Corresponding author.
E-mail address: pkkokota@pediatrics.wisc.edu (P. K. Kokotailo).

MI has often been associated with the transtheoretical model or stages of change model in which behavior change is viewed as a process of stage of readiness.[3] Readiness to change may fluctuate, and an adolescent may change stages over the course of an office visit, or not for months or years. The health care provider can be a facilitator or a barrier to behavior change depending on how well he or she matches counseling to the patient's stage of readiness to change. MI seems to be particularly effective for those who are not interested in change (precontemplation stage) or are thinking about change but are not yet prepared to make a commitment (contemplation stage). The determination/preparation stage is that in which the individual is firmly committed to making immediate change, usually within 1 month. Action stage is the stage in which behavior change has already begun but is not yet a habitual pattern, and maintenance stage is that in which a behavior change is well established, typically for 6 months or longer. During relapse, or resumption of an unhealthy behavior, MI can be used to reframe relapse as a normal part of the change process and as a learning opportunity that leads to reassessing readiness to change. Although these steps may follow sequentially, an adolescent may move between stages and back quite easily (see Fig 1).

THE SPIRIT OF MI

MI is a style of communication rather than a group of techniques. The key features of the spirit of MI are collaboration, evocation, and autonomy. "Collaboration" is a partnership that is created between the health care provider and

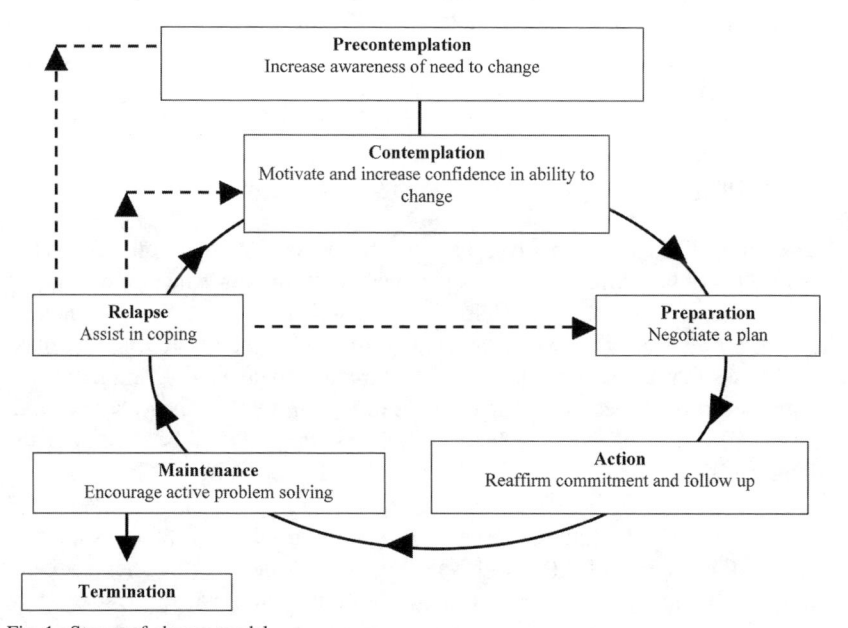

Fig 1. Stages of change model.

the adolescent. The patient's perspectives are respected and valued by the provider. "Evocation" is when the health care provider facilitates exploration of reasons for and against change by eliciting the adolescent's intrinsic motivation for change by using open-ended questions and reflections. Motivation to change is elicited from the adolescent, not imposed by the health care provider. The health care provider is directive in helping the adolescent examine and eventually resolve ambivalence regarding values, goals, beliefs, and current behavior. "Autonomy" is when the health care provider acknowledges that the choice to make change resides with the adolescent. The adolescent will decide if, how, and when behavior change will occur, and although the provider guides the decision, direct persuasion is not used.

Four fundamental principles are the basis of MI: (1) expressing empathy; (2) developing discrepancy; (3) rolling with resistance; and (4) supporting self-efficacy.

When providers express empathy by accepting patients' beliefs and behaviors, even those that may be unhealthy, they facilitate behavior change. In contrast, resistance to change often arises when providers apply pressure by attempting to directly persuade and rationalize why the individual should change. Adolescents, especially those who have an oppositional or defiant temperament, often respond to authoritarian styles characterized by persuasion and pressure by pushing back rather than considering change. With the use of empathy, an atmosphere of safety is created that allows the adolescent to talk about activities and beliefs without judgment, and this setting promotes self-focus and self-disclosure. The use of reflective listening can aid in promoting disclosure as well. Even when dealing with more concerning health behaviors, the health care provider can be more effective by resisting giving advice until it is requested or the provider has specifically asked the adolescent's permission to share his or her perspective. This eliciting, nonpressuring, empathic style is often in contrast to other interpersonal interactions that the adolescent has experienced with other adults and may encourage a therapeutic alliance with the health care provider.

Developing discrepancy involves eliciting from the adolescent any difference between his or her current status and personal goals, or between current behavior and personal values or beliefs. Helping the adolescent become aware of internal inconsistencies usually provokes an attempt to resolve the discrepancy by making changes that are more consistent with personal goals, values, and beliefs. A health care provider can offer objective information that can be valuable feedback needed to recognize discrepancies, but this must always be done with the adolescent's permission.

Avoiding arguments with an adolescent by rolling with resistance is another important principle of MI. Ambivalence about whether to change an unhealthy behavior is normal, and arguing with an individual to persuade him or her to change is generally counterproductive. Resistance occurs when the health care provider and adolescent do not see eye-to-eye on an issue, and usually the adolescent feels pushed to do something he or she is not yet ready to do. The health care provider and the adolescent are mismatched in where they see the adolescent's stage of readiness to change. Resistance is a reflection of intrapersonal or interpersonal ambivalence and can be depicted by signs such as arguing, interrupting, missing appointments, and not performing requested tasks such as keeping a symptom diary. Some adolescents may also express resistance by being "too compliant," by agreeing too easily with everything the provider suggests. When resistance is recognized, it is a signal to the health care provider to change strategies.

The last principle of MI is to support self-efficacy. Despair or denial of a problem may occur when an individual lacks confidence in his or her ability to change a situation. A provider may help support an adolescent's ability to make a change successfully by expressing optimism about the possibility of change and provide hope by reframing change as a gradual, stepwise process and not an all-or-nothing venture. Helping adolescents to identify a range of effective alternatives for achieving a goal is one way to support self-efficacy, as is helping the adolescent to identify past successes and reframe previous failures as learning opportunities.

STRATEGIES FOR ESTABLISHING RAPPORT

There are 4 strategies in MI that help develop rapport between a patient and a health care provider: (1) open-ended questions; (2) affirmations; (3) reflective listening; and (4) summaries.

Open-ended questions are those that cannot be answered with "yes/no" or a short 1- or 2-word answer such as "nothing," and they encourage adolescents to express their thoughts, feelings, and issues. Examples include "What concerns do you have today?" and "Tell me about your smoking." With younger adolescents, it may be more developmentally appropriate to give some choices first ("Would you like to talk about your weight or your grades in school today?"), but always end with an open-ended question ("What would you like to discuss today?").

Reflective listening is a statement of understanding of an adolescent's experience, communicated nonjudgmentally. Simple and complex reflections may be used. Simple reflections are an accurate reflection of what the adolescent just said, whereas a complex reflection is an expansion on the meaning or intent of what the adolescent said.

Affirmations are statements of appreciation for the adolescent's efforts or participation such as saying, "Thanks for working with me today. You have some excellent ideas." or "Honesty is really important. I'm glad you could tell me about that."

Summaries bring together what the adolescent has previously expressed and may include some basic interpretation of the issues. Three types of summaries include: collecting summaries that replay several previously expressed ideas or feelings; linking summaries that connect several previously expressed ideas or feelings the adolescent had not connected together; and transitional summaries that combine essential components of the preceding discussion in preparation for a shift in the focus of the discussion.

TECHNIQUES AND STRATEGIES USED IN MI

There are 7 strategies used in MI and behavior-change counseling: (1) asking permission; (2) using elicit-provide-elicit; (3) using a decisional balance; (4) using importance and confidence rulers; (5) agenda setting; (6) using the "FRAMES" paragraph; and (7) using a behavior-change worksheet. Each strategy can be used to increase rapport or build motivation for change.

1. Asking permission: Before offering information or advice, the health care provider can assess whether the adolescent would like new information or suggestions by asking permission:

    "Would it be okay if I told you what I think about this?"

    "Some of my patients have told me that __ has been helpful to them when they have been in your situation. May I tell you what they found?"

    If permission is asked and the adolescent declines information or advice, the health care provider should be respectful and move on to another topic that the adolescent might be more interested in discussing.

2. Using elicit-provide-elicit for information and advice: An approach that can save time and build rapport is to first elicit what the adolescent already knows about a topic and/or options for behavior change. Often, the adolescent already has the knowledge or has excellent ideas regarding what to do. The provider can then assist the adolescent in making a plan that is realistic and successful rather than expending time and energy providing unneeded information or advice. When information is missing or inaccurate or when the provider thinks providing information or advice might be helpful, permission to give the information or advice should be requested. After providing information or advice, it is most important to again elicit the adolescent's reaction to what has been said by asking, "What do you make of this information or these options? How does this change things for you?"

3. Using decisional balance: Asking the adolescent about his or her own perceived pros and cons regarding change can also help motivate a behavior

change. Phrasing can help; asking about the "good" and "not-so-good" things about change rather than the "good" and the "bad" aspects is less threatening and more likely to encourage disclosure on both sides. For an individual in the precontemplation stage, it may be most helpful to ask about the pros first, followed by the cons, of keeping things the same. When an adolescent is contemplating change, it may be more productive to ask about pros first, followed by the cons, of change, as illustrated below. After eliciting the adolescent's perception of both sides of the decisional balance, the provider can summarize the 2 sides, always presenting the adolescent's own arguments for change second, followed by an open-ended question prompting for change or commitment talk. For example, one can say, "Some of the good things about having sex without a condom are ___, and at the same time, some of the not-so-good things about having sex without a condom are ___. So how do you feel about this now?"

4. Using importance and confidence rulers: Another MI strategy is to assess the level of importance and confidence to make a behavior change and determine whether to focus on reasons to change or confidence in ability to change. One can ask, "On a scale from 0 to 10, where 10 is the most important and 0 is the least important, what number would you give for how important it is to you to [behavior change] right now? Why is it a [current number] instead of a [lower number]? What would need to happen to make it a [higher number]?" Then ask, "On a scale from 0 to 10, where 10 is the most confident and 0 is the least confident, what number would you give for how confident you are that you could [behavior change] if you wanted to right now? Why is it a [current number] instead of a [lower number]? What would need to happen to make it a [higher number]?"

Some adolescents have difficulty using numbers to signify an ordinal scale without a visual aid. A helpful adaptation is to draw 2 separate visual scales such as those shown in Fig 2.

Ask the adolescent to point on each scale to indicate how important and how confident he or she feels about making a specific behavior change.

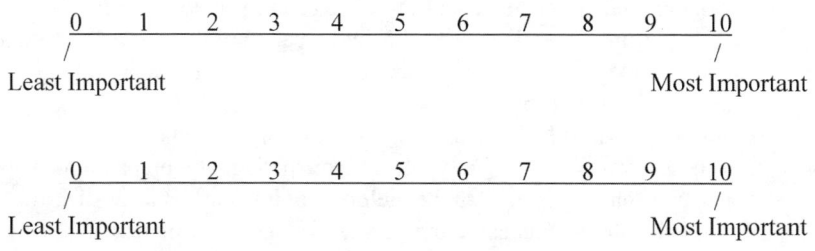

```
    0   1   2   3   4   5   6   7   8   9   10
    /                                         /
Least Important                     Most Important


    0   1   2   3   4   5   6   7   8   9   10
    /                                         /
Least Important                     Most Important
```

Fig 2. Sample visual scales.

The focus of the conversation will depend on the rating levels for importance and confidence. If one number is distinctly lower than the other, focus on the lower number first. If importance is low (≤5) or if both importance and confidence levels are about the same, focus on importance. If both are very low (≤3), explore feelings about talking about the behavior.

If the focus is on importance, ask, "What made you choose [current number] and not a lower number? What makes [behavior] this important?" Reflect reasons given and ask for elaboration: "Tell me more about that." Then, ask for more reasons by saying, "What else makes it important?" and summarize by saying, "So what makes this important right now? What would have to happen for [behavior] to be a little bit more important to you?" Reflect and ask for elaboration by saying "What else?" Then summarize by saying, "So what makes [behavior change] important is ___, and at the same time [behavior change] would be more important to you if ___."

If the focus is on confidence, ask: "What made you choose [current number] and not a lower number? What makes you feel this confident that you can [behavior]?" Reflect reasons given and ask for elaboration: "Tell me more about that." Then, ask for more reasons by saying "What else makes you feel confident?" and summarize by saying, "So what makes you feel confident that you can [behavior] right now is ___." Then ask, "What would have to happen for you to feel a little bit more confident that you can [behavior]?" Reflect and ask for elaboration by saying, "what else?" Then summarize by saying, "So what makes you confident that you can [behavior] is ___. You would feel more confident about [behavior] if ___."

5. Agenda setting: When more than one health behavior is identified that could benefit from change, setting an agenda helps to efficiently prioritize and focus the discussion on the one behavior in which the adolescent is most interested and agrees to target. The goal of agenda setting is for the provider to understand the adolescent's agenda and let the adolescent select a behavior to discuss, although negotiation to discuss a provider's concern can also be included. An adolescent is more likely to change a behavior when he or she selects the focus. Charts with a number of behaviors depicted may aid in prioritizing the behavior to choose.
6. Using the FRAMES paragraph: The acronym FRAMES (feedback, responsibility, advice, menu of options, empathy, and self-efficacy) has been used to describe the 6 components of effective brief intervention (see Table 1). One way of incorporating FRAMES into a patient interaction is to formulate a FRAMES paragraph at the end of the visit, incorporating the elements noted in Table 1.
7. Using a behavior-change plan: On the basis of the adolescent's stage of readiness to change, especially when he or she is in the preparation stage, a behavior-change plan can be helpful to implement ideas that were discussed. Adolescents can either develop a plan with the assistance of a

Table 1
FRAMES: elements of effective brief intervention

Element	Description	Effect
Feedback	Provide, in an objective, noncoercive manner, personalized information regarding the risks or consequences associated with the current behavior or state (best done after eliciting permission to provide feedback and getting an affirmative response).	Raises awareness of negative consequences, increases problem recognition, and "develops discrepancy" between actual and ideal circumstances while communicating attentiveness and interest.
Responsibility	Communicate that any decision about whether to change is solely the adolescent's decision and that change will only occur if he or she chooses to take the steps necessary to accomplish it.	Minimizes reactivity; supports sense of autonomy; paves way for offering expert perspective.
Advice	Offer, in a concerned and supportive manner, a clear recommendation that the adolescent make a change (best done after eliciting permission to provide advice and getting an affirmative response).	Provides sense of comfort, direction, or inspiration from expert guidance.
Menu of options	Offer a range of alternatives for how to accomplish the desired goal and engage the teen in actively weighing the options to determine which would be the best "fit" (best done after eliciting the adolescent's own ideas).	Increases likelihood of keeping commitment; enhances sense of freedom and control; provides concrete assistance in changing.
Empathy	Communicate accurate understanding of the adolescent's experience (thoughts, feelings, wishes, fears) in a warm, nonjudgmental manner.	Builds alliance; creates "atmosphere of safety"; promotes disclosure; clarifies adolescent's perceptions.
Self-efficacy	Support the adolescent's belief in his or her own ability to succeed at change and communicate optimism about the prospects for doing so.	Prevents defensive or hopeless reactions to problem recognition; enhances confidence and willingness to attempt new behaviors.

Adapted from Bien TH, Miller WR, Tonigan JS. Addiction. *1993;88(3):315–336 (see also Miller WR, Rollnick S.* Motivational Interviewing: Preparing People to Change Addictive Behavior. *New York, NY: Guilford Press; 1991).*

health care provider or on their own. A typical behavior-change plan includes the following components:

- The changes I want to make are ___.
- The most important reason I want to make these changes are ___.
- The specific steps I plan to make in changing are ___.
- Some people who can support are ___. Here is how they can help: ___.
- How I will know my plan is working: ___.
- Things that could interfere with my plan (barriers) and possible solutions: ___.

The critical components of negotiating a plan are to set concrete and specific goals by (1) using elicit-provide-elicit, (2) addressing obstacles and eliciting or providing solutions, (3) eliciting commitment, and (4) arranging for follow-up. The plan should be specific, measurable, achievable, realistic, and time-framed.

EVIDENCE FOR MI AS AN EFFECTIVE COUNSELING STRATEGY FOR ADOLESCENTS

Most of the early work in evaluating the effects of using MI as a counseling style was performed with adults and, initially, in the area of alcohol and other drug abuse. It has often been difficult to study the effects of motivational techniques, because the studies often included MI as a component in a complex intervention, and especially in earlier work, interventions may not have been standardized with intervention providers who adhered faithfully to the spirit of MI.[4,5] Over the past decade, the method has been evaluated in many areas including addiction, smoking cessation, weight loss, changing physical activity, asthma treatment, diabetes treatment, and adherence to treatment.[6] Scientific methodology has improved, and training of providers has become more standardized and shown to be effective in having practitioners adhere to MI methods as well as influence their professional behavior.[7-10] It has been shown in several large reviews that adaptations of MI are generally more effective in changing single behaviors than no or minimal treatment and are usually as effective as more intensive alternative treatments.[6,11-13]

Has MI been shown to be effective in changing behaviors in adolescents? There are more studies recently that examined changes in health behaviors such as those associated with eating disorders, diabetes care, improving nutrition, weight loss, and decreasing risky sexual behaviors in adolescents, but the most research has been performed in relation to alcohol, tobacco, and other drug use in youth. Studies involving alcohol use include an early study by Monti et al,[14] who showed that alcohol-using 18- to 19-year-old adolescents who received an MI intervention in a hospital emergency department displayed equivalent levels of alcohol-use reduction compared with a standard-hospital-care group. At a 6-month follow-up, however, the MI group showed decreased harmful behaviors, including decreased episodes of drinking and driving, alcohol-related injuries, and other alcohol-related problems when compared with the standard-care group. In a review of Department of Motor Vehicle records, those in the MI group were significantly less likely to have a moving violation in the 6 months after treatment than those in the standard-care group. Spirito et al[15] studied 13- to 17-year-old alcohol-using youth who were randomly assigned to receive either MI or standard emergency department care and found that both groups showed decreased quantity of drinking at the 12-month follow-up. At the 12-month follow-up, adolescents who screened positive for problematic use at baseline reported significantly more improvement on 2 of 3 alcohol-use outcomes if they received MI compared with standard care. Baer et al[16] found similar results with college freshman who reported heavy drinking while in high school who received a single-session, preventive MI-based intervention. When compared with a high-risk control group in this randomized trial, at the 4-year follow-up there were significant reductions for the intervention group in quantity and frequency of alcohol use, but the magnitude of change was greatest for reduction of negative drinking consequences. Another randomized, controlled trial examined the effects of a single MI-based intervention on use of contraception and use of alcohol in college-aged young women.[17] In this study, the intervention group showed increased effective contraception use and decreased risky drinking compared with controls at the 1-month follow-up.

A recent Cochrane systematic review[18] of primary prevention for alcohol misuse in young people revealed many limitations in the design and methodology of primary prevention programs, including many different theoretical perspectives and settings for programs, use of a range of different outcome measures, and poor quality of much research on the effectiveness of interventions. Studies by Monti et al[14] (see above) and Marlatt[19] (a preceding study to that of Baer et al[16]) included in the review were noted to have "strong design with strong analysis" and "strong design and consistent pattern of results indicating potential value of motivational interviewing," respectively.

One of the best evaluations of the effect of MI on drug-use prevention for young people <25 years old in nonschool settings was performed by Gates et al[20] for the Cochrane Database of Systematic Reviews in 2006. In this systematic review, 17 studies were included to evaluate 4 types of intervention, including brief intervention/MI. Two studies that used MI were reviewed. Thirty-two studies were excluded from review, with many of these randomized, controlled trials being affected by methodologic problems, with especially high levels of loss to follow-up. Review included too few studies for firm conclusions, but one study of MI suggested that this intervention may be beneficial in preventing cannabis use.[21]

The Cannabis Youth Treatment Study[22] also examined the effectiveness and cost-effectiveness of two interrelated randomized trials that studied 5 short-term interventions for youth with cannabis-use disorders. MET plus cognitive behavioral therapy was 1 of the therapies used, and the results showed that all 5 interventions demonstrated significant treatment effects during the 12 months after random assignment to a treatment intervention. Treatment including MET was considered one of the most cost-effective interventions.

Grimshaw and Stanton,[4] in a Cochrane review, also studied tobacco-cessation interventions for young people in 2006. Of the 15 studies that satisfied the inclusion criteria for the review, 3 studies were based on interventions that targeted the stage of change of individuals using the transtheoretical model, and 9 studies used some form of motivational enhancement for young people. Three studies used MI as a component of the intervention. A number of interventions used a combination of methods. The reviewers concluded that the trials that evaluated the transtheoretical model achieved moderate long-term success, with a pooled odds ratio at one year of 1.7 (95% confidence interval: 1.25–2.33) and a 2-year follow-up odds ratio of 1.38 (95% confidence interval: 0.99–1.92). It was felt that it was impossible to isolate the effect of the MI in the 3 interventions reviewed, because not all 3 trials studied MI alone, and it was felt that it was inappropriate to disaggregate the effectiveness of a single component in different complex interventions. When the odds ratios for these 3 trials were pooled, however, the odds ratio was 2.05 (95% confidence interval: 1.10–3.80). The review authors concluded that there was not yet sufficient evidence to support the effectiveness of smoking-cessation programs for adolescents, although some approaches, including those tailored to an adolescent's preparation for quitting and behavioral therapy programs, have shown promise.

Other studies have investigated behavioral change in adolescents and young adults through the use of MI in other areas such as increasing fruit and vegetable consumption, reducing sexual risk, achieving better diabetes mellitus control, reducing lipid levels, preventing and treating obesity, and treating eating disorders.[23–28] Although methodologic problems still persist, it appears that MI has been at least partially effective in managing these behavioral issues. Significant behavior change has also been demonstrated with the use of MI in conjunction with other methods, such as stage-of-change–based newsletters and computer-based communication with individually tailored e-mail follow-up[23]. Using MI with other methods may be practical as a relatively inexpensive approach and one that could be used with more geographically dispersed populations.

CONCLUSIONS AND IMPLICATIONS

MI and behavior-change counseling may be particularly appropriate with adolescents. Adolescents are often in an exploratory phase of risk-taking behaviors, and using MI may be very effective in these precontemplative and contemplative stages. Adolescents who are struggling to become independent may often exhibit resistance to adult authority figures, and the patient-centered style used with MI, including "rolling with resistance," may fit well in helping adolescents feel that they have more control in their lives. Because adolescents have little patience for dealing with issues in which they have no interest, MI is developmentally appropriate and can be tailored to their unique needs, feelings, circumstances, and readiness to change.[26]

Although the use of formal MI may go beyond what a health care provider can do in a relatively short medical encounter, using the style of MI and conveying its spirit of negotiation and collaboration in health care is most important. The use of MI style and strategies can support adolescent autonomy and make clinical encounters more enjoyable for both the adolescent and practitioner. Although many patients report higher satisfaction from patient-centered communication in medical practice,[29] there are also individuals who prefer a more directive approach.[30] As with many areas of adolescent medicine, it is beneficial for medical providers to be flexible in their communication style and attentive to shifting patient needs.

Rollnick et al[13] eloquently advocated for a flexible guiding style in patient encounters that involve behavior change. He described the guiding style as a simplified form of MI in which a practitioner steps aside from persuasion and instead encourages patients to explore their own motivations and aspirations. Although the core skills of asking, informing, and listening are used in both directive and guiding encounters, in the directing style, informing is usually the dominant mode. In the guiding style, asking involves eliciting from patients how or why they might change. Informing is combined with asking to encourage choice of behaviors and promote autonomy rather than the doctor telling the patient what to do. Listening is used to convey understanding of patient experiences and encourage further patient exploration as to how he or she might change behavior. It may be difficult at first for a doctor or other health care provider to restrain himself or herself and hand over the responsibility and choice to the patient rather than "fixing it." Guiding, however, may promote less resistance and promote alliance with a young person. Shifting back and forth from the directing to guiding style may also be necessary, even within the same visit.

Evidence of effectiveness of MI and adaptations of MI have varied, as noted above, but the evidence continues to mount in favor of using the MI style with adolescents in many areas of behavior change.[10,27,31,32] Future directions for research in MI include the use of larger and more diverse samples for study of health behaviors. There is a need for more detailed and rigorous intervention approaches to ensure intervention fidelity. Intervention fidelity is complicated by the considerable variability in the way that MI is conceptualized as well as delivered and assessed across studies. Another important area of study is the examination of the extent to which the effects of MI are attributable to MI itself as opposed to the more generic aspects of counseling such as empathy and attention to the individual.[27] Additional areas of research may include how to most beneficially involve parents in behavior-change consultations, maximize access to MI through computer-based and computer-assisted interventions, and study the effect of MI with other interventions such as cognitive behavioral therapy and narrative therapy. Research in cost-effectiveness of interventions will also be important. Improved methodologic rigor in research will be important for all of these areas of research, including long-term follow-up of participants.

Resources for health care providers who want to increase their skills in MI include the use of books and articles. Good detailed examples of MI and behavior-change counseling including phrases to incorporate into encounters are available in written formats,[26,33–36] CDs and DVDs,[37–39] and Web-based material.[40] The Web site www.motivationalinterview.org includes references involving all media and a compendium of training opportunities for health care professionals.

REFERENCES

1. Miller WR, Rollnick S. *Motivational Interviewing: Preparing People for Change.* 2nd ed. New York, NY: Guilford Press; 2002
2. Miller WR, Zweben A, DiClemente CC, Rychtarik RG. *Motivational Enhancement Therapy Manual: A Clinical Research Guide for Therapists Treating Individuals With Alcohol Abuse and Dependence.* Rockville, MD: National Institute on Alcohol Abuse and Alcoholism; 1992
3. Prochaska JO, DiClemente CC. Transtheoretical therapy: toward a more integrative model of change. *Psychother Theory Res Pract.* 1982;19(3):276–288
4. Grimshaw GM, Stanton A. Tobacco cessation interventions for young people. *Cochrane Database Syst Rev.* 2006;(4):CD003289
5. Tevyaw TO, Monti PM. Motivational enhancement and other brief interventions for adolescent substance abuse: foundations, applications and evaluation. *Addiction.* 2004;99(suppl 2):63–75
6. Rubak S, Sandbaek A, Lauritzen T, Christensen B. Motivational interviewing: a systematic review and meta-analysis. *Br J Gen Pract.* 2005;55(513):305–312
7. Schoener EP, Madeja CL, Henderson MJ, Ondersma SJ, Janisse JJ. Effects of motivational interviewing training on mental health therapist behavior. *Drug Alcohol Depend.* 2006;82(3):269–275
8. Baer JS, Rosengren DB, Dunn CW, Wells EA, Ogle RL, Hartzler B. An evaluation of workshop training in motivational interviewing for addiction and mental health clinicians. *Drug Alcohol Depend.* 2004;73(1):99–106
9. Tober G, Godfrey C, Parrott S, et al. Setting standards for training and competence: the UK alcohol treatment trial. *Alcohol Alcohol.* 2005;40(5):413–418
10. Rubak S, Sandbaek A, Lauritzen T, Borch-Johnsen K, Christensen B. An education and training course in motivational interviewing influence: GPs' professional behaviour—ADDITION Denmark. *Br J Gen Pract.* 2006;56(527):429–436
11. Burke BL, Arkowitz H, Menchoa M. The efficacy of motivational interviewing: a meta-analysis of controlled clinical trials. *J Consult Clin Psychol.* 2003;71(5):843–861
12. Britt E, Hudson S, Blampied N. Motivational interviewing in health settings: a review. *Patient Educ Couns.* 2004;53(2):147–155
13. Rollnick S, Butler CC, McCambridge J, Kinnersley P, Elwyn G, Resnicow K. Consultations about changing behaviour. *BMJ.* 2005;331(7522):961–963

14. Monti PM, Spirito A, Myers M, et al. Brief intervention for harm reduction with alcohol-positive older adolescents in a hospital emergency department. *J Consult Clin Psychol.* 1999;67(6):989–994
15. Spirito A, Monti PM, Barnett NP, et al. A randomized clinical trial of a brief motivational intervention for alcohol-positive adolescents treated in an emergency department. *J Pediatr.* 2004;145(3):396–402
16. Baer JS, Kivlahan DR, Blume AW, McKnight P, Marlatt GA. Brief intervention for heavy-drinking college students: 4-year follow-up and natural history. *Am J Public Health.* 2001;91(8):1310–1316
17. Ingersoll KS, Ceperich SD, Nettleman MD, Karanda K, Brocksen S, Johnson BA. Reducing alcohol-exposed pregnancy risk in college women: Initial outcomes of a clinical trial of a motivational intervention. *J Subst Abuse Treat.* 2005;29(3):173–180
18. Foxcroft DR, Ireland D, Lister-Sharp DJ, Lowe G, Breen R. Primary prevention for alcohol misuse in young people. *Cochrane Database Syst Rev.* 2002;(3):CD003024
19. Marlatt GA, Baer JS, Kivlahan DR, et al. Screening and brief intervention for high-risk college student drinkers: results from a 2-year follow-up assessment. *J Consult Clin Psychol.* 1998;66(4):604–615
20. Gates S, McCambridge J, Smith LA, Foxcroft DR. Interventions for prevention of drug use by young people delivered in non-school settings. *Cochrane Database Syst Rev.* 2006;(1):CD005030
21. McCambridge J, Strang J. The efficacy of single-session motivational interviewing in reducing drug consumption and perceptions of drug-related risk and harm among young people: results from a multi-site cluster randomized trial. *Addiction.* 2004;99(1):39–52
22. Dennis M, Godley SH, Diamond G, et al. The Cannabis Youth Treatment (CYT) Study: main findings from two randomized trials. *J Subst Abuse Treat.* 2004;27(3):197–213
23. Richards A, Kattelmann KK, Ren C. Motivating 18- to 24-year-olds to increase their fruit and vegetable consumption. *J Am Diet Assoc.* 2006;106(9):1405–1411
24. Kiene SM, Barta WD. A brief individualized computer-delivered sexual risk reduction intervention increases HIV/AIDS preventive behavior. *J Adolesc Health.* 2006;39(3):404–410
25. Channon S, Smith VJ, Gregory JW. A pilot study of motivational interviewing in adolescents with diabetes. *Arch Dis Child.* 2003;88(8):680–683
26. Berg-Smith S, Stevens V, Brown K, et al. A brief motivational intervention to improve dietary adherence in adolescents. The Dietary Intervention Study in Children (DISC) Research Group. *Health Educ Res.* 1999;14(3):399–341
27. Resnicow K, Davis R, Rollnick S. Motivational interviewing for pediatric obesity: conceptual issues and evidence review. *J Am Diet Assoc.* 2006;106(12):2024–2033
28. Kotler LA, Boudreau GS, Devlin MJ. Emerging psychotherapies for eating disorders. *J Psychiatr Pract.* 2003;9(6):431–441
29. Wanzer MB, Booth-Butterfiels M, Gruber K. Perceptions of health care providers' communication: relationships between patient-centered communication and satisfaction. *Health Commun.* 2004;16(3):363–383
30. Swenson SL, Buell S, Zettler P, White M, Ruston DC, Lo B. Patient-centered communication: do patients really prefer it? *J Gen Intern Med.* 2004;19(11):1069–1079
31. Erickson SJ, Gerstle M, Feldstein SW. Brief interventions and motivational interviewing with children, adolescents, and their parents in pediatric health care settings: a review. *Arch Pediatr Adolesc Med.* 2005;159(12):1173–1180
32. Sindelar HA, Abrantes AM, Hart C, Lewander W, Spirito A. Motivational interviewing in pediatric practice. *Curr Probl Pediatr Adolesc Health Care.* 2004;34(9):322–339
33. Gold MA, Hatcher RA, Horwitz M, Greene A, Taleb S. *Teen to Teen: Plain Talk From Teens About Sex, Self-esteem and Everything in Between.* Dawsonville, GA: Bridging the Gap Communications; 2005:9–11
34. Rollnick S, Mason P, Butler C. *Health Behavior Change: A Guide for Practitioners.* London, United Kingdom: Churchill Livingstone; 1999

35. Conard LE, Gold MA. Emergency contraception update: providing emergency contraception in the pediatrician's office. *Contemp Pediatr.* 2006;23(2):49–70
36. Ott MA, Labbett RL, Gold MA. Counseling adolescents about abstinence in the office setting. *J Pediatr Adolesc Gynecol.* 2007;20(1):39–44
37. Allison J. *MI in Practice: The Edinburgh Interview 2006* [CD-ROM]. Jeff Allison Training Ltd, UK; 2006. Available at: www.jeffallison.co.uk/training_materials.html. Accessed March 11, 2008
38. Gilligan T, Mason P. *Engaging Motivation* [DVD or VHS video]. Pip Mason Consultancy Ltd, UK; 2006. Available at www.pipmason.com/publications/training_materials.aspx. Accessed March 11, 2008
39. Miller WR, Rollnick S, Moyers TB. *Motivational Interviewing: Professional Training Series* [DVD or VHS video]. University of New Mexico, Albuquerque, NM; 1998. Available at: http://motivationalinterview.org/training/videos.html.
40. Gold MA. Case commentary: gynecological care for adolescents. *Virtual Mentor.* 2003;5(5). Available at: http://virtualmentor.ama-assn.org/2003/05/ccas1-0305.html. Accessed March 5, 2008

Motivational Interviewing and Sexual and Contraceptive Behaviors

Melanie A. Gold, DO[a]*, Kristin Delisi, MSN, CRNP[b]

[a]*Division of Adolescent Medicine, Department of Pediatrics, University of Pittsburgh School of Medicine, Medical Arts Building, Suite 500.9, 3708 Fifth Avenue, Pittsburgh, PA 15213, USA*

[b]*Division of Adolescent Medicine, Children's Hospital of Pittsburgh, University of Pittsburgh Medical Center, 3705 Fifth Avenue, Pittsburgh, PA 15213, USA*

Motivational interviewing (MI) has been described by Petersen et al[1] as a promising way to address women's risk-taking behaviors. They proposed using MI to counsel about contraception, specifically by exploring discrepancies between pregnancy intention and contraceptive use and between sexually transmitted disease (STD) risk and condom use. They also suggested using MI to share information and promote behaviors to reduce risk. To date, most MI interventions related to pregnancy have been aimed at reducing tobacco and alcohol use by adult pregnant women.[2–13] There have been 2 studies that assessed the impact of MI on preventing pregnancy, but none have assessed the impact of MI on preventing both pregnancy and STDs, and none have included women under the age of 18 years or men. The 2 studies that assessed MI related to preventing pregnancy focused on reducing risk of alcohol-exposed pregnancy (AEP) rather than on preventing unintended pregnancy in general. Ingersoll et al[14] tested the feasibility and impact of MI in reducing drinking and/or increasing effective contraception use in 190 women who were at risk for an AEP in a multisite single-arm pilot study at 6 community settings in 3 large cities. The intervention consisted of 4 manual-guided motivational counseling sessions and 1 contraceptive counseling session. Among 143 women who completed follow-up (75.3% of the original sample), 68.5% were no longer at risk for an AEP, 12.6% reduced their drinking only, 23.1% used effective contraception only, and 32.9% changed both behaviors. Results were consistent across all 6 diverse high-risk community settings. This study provided support for the feasibility and potential impact of MI conducted in community settings to change contraceptive behaviors. In 2005, Ingersoll et al[15] conducted a randomized, controlled trial of a single-session MI-based intervention to reduce AEP risk among college women. Among 228 women aged 18 to 24 years who were at risk for an AEP, 15% of the control

*Corresponding author.
E-mail address: magold@pitt.edu (M. A. Gold).

Copyright © 2008 American Academy of Pediatrics. All rights reserved. ISSN 1934-4287

group and 25% of the MI group reported no risk drinking at the 1-month follow-up. Significantly fewer women in the control group (48%) used effective contraception at follow-up compared with those in the MI group (64%), and significantly more women in the MI group (74%) were no longer at risk for an AEP compared with those in the control group (54%). This study demonstrated the efficacy of a single session of MI in improving contraceptive behaviors.

MI has been described as a way to counsel adolescents about sexual abstinence and emergency contraception.[16,17] MI techniques such as open-ended questions, affirmations, reflections, and summaries enhance rapport and improve discussions about adolescents' beliefs and intentions regarding contraception and STD prevention. Conard and Gold[17] described how these techniques can be used to help clinicians assess an adolescent's level of knowledge about emergency contraception. This patient-centered approach helps adolescents learn important information regarding contraception to make informed decisions.

OVERVIEW

Strategies from MI can be adapted to address both sexual and contraceptive behaviors. Techniques such as agenda setting and assessing readiness to change can be used to define which sexual or contraceptive behaviors the adolescent wishes to discuss and how ready an adolescent is to change a health behavior. Assessing readiness to change and matching counseling strategy to readiness to change is a critical aspect of any reproductive health visit. MI spirit and style can enhance youth receptivity to information and advice that the clinician may wish to offer.

OPENING STRATEGIES

Four strategies in MI help develop rapport between an adolescent and a health care provider: (1) using open-ended questions; (2) providing affirmations; (3) practicing reflective listening; and (4) using summaries.

Open-Ended Questions

Open-ended questions are those that encourage adolescents to express their thoughts, feelings, and issues. A particularly helpful open-ended question to use during a reproductive health visit is, "How old do you want to be when you have your first [next] baby? Why then and not now?" Assuming that the adolescent states an age that is older than he or she is currently, these open-ended questions encourage adolescents to talk about reasons for delaying pregnancy. Whenever possible, encourage both male and female adolescents to talk about the positive goals and future they envision rather than simply reporting wanting to avoid negative consequences such as not wanting to get pregnant or to avoid STDs. Individuals are more likely to move toward change when they strive for positive goals and rewards rather than to solely avoid negative consequences or punishments. Another helpful open-ended question that can elicit adolescents' perspectives is to say, "Tell me how you feel about becoming [or remaining] sexually active. What would be [or is] good about it? What would be [or is] not so good about it? How do you see it?" With younger adolescents, it is more developmentally appropriate to give some closed-ended choices first such as, "Would you like to talk about ways to prevent pregnancy, or how to avoid STDs, or ways to stay abstinent today?" Always end with an open-ended question such as, "What would you like to discuss today?"

Affirmations

Affirmations are statements of appreciation or compliments for the adolescent's knowledge, efforts, or participation. Examples include: "Thank you for discussing this with me today. You have some excellent ideas," "You really know what birth control method will work for you," "That's a great idea to always keep condoms in your purse so you have them when you need them," "You know a lot about different birth control options and seem to be choosing carefully what you know will work best for you," "I appreciate your being honest with me that you are having trouble remembering to take the pill," and "I respect the fact that you can tell me honestly what you do and do not want to talk about."

Reflections

Reflections are statements that demonstrate health care providers' understanding of each adolescent's experiences and feelings; they are communicated in a nonjudgmental manner. Simple reflections are an accurate statement of what the adolescent just said in the form of repetition or a paraphrase, whereas complex reflections expand on the meaning or intent of what the adolescent said. Table 1 shows some examples of reflections that could be used in a reproductive health setting.

Summaries

Summaries pull together what the adolescent has previously said during the visit and may include some basic interpretation of the issues. Three types of summaries used in reproductive health visits are: (1) collecting summaries that replay several previously expressed ideas or feelings related to pregnancy, abstinence, or STD experiences; (2) linking summaries that connect several previously expressed ideas or feelings that the adolescent had not connected together (such as recalling his or her distress over a pregnancy scare while discussing what is most important in choosing a contraceptive method); and (3) using transitional summaries that combine essential components of the preceding discussion. These summaries prepare for a shift in the focus of the discussion to decide if the adolescent wants to initiate a change in behavior such as abstinence, starting a new contraceptive method, or switching methods.

Table 1
Examples of reflections that could be used in a reproductive health setting

Type of Reflection	Description	Example
Simple reflection	Say back to the adolescent what he or she has just said, staying close to his or her words.	Adolescent: "You say that I should use something to keep from getting pregnant, but I don't think I need it. I have unprotected sex all the time and I haven't gotten pregnant!" Clinician: "You're not sure that using birth control is really necessary because you haven't gotten pregnant after having unprotected sex in the past."
Reflection of meaning	Reflect the implied or underlying meaning of what the adolescent just said.	Adolescent: "You say that I should use something to keep from getting pregnant, but I don't think I need it. I have unprotected sex all the time and I haven't gotten pregnant!" Clinician: "You think there is something wrong and you can't get pregnant."
Reflection of feeling	Reflect the implied or underlying feelings behind what was said.	Adolescent: "You say that I should use something to keep from getting pregnant, but I don't think I need it. I have unprotected sex all the time and I haven't gotten pregnant!" Clinician: "It worries you that you might not be able to get pregnant when you want to."
Double-sided reflection	Use when both sides of ambivalence have been expressed; reflect both perspectives, usually starting with the side that favors the status quo and ending with the side that favors change.	Adolescent: "Sometimes I get mad at myself for not using condoms every time we have sex, but I only have sex with one person, so I know I won't get an STD." Clinician: "You don't believe that you're at risk of getting an STD, and at the same time it bothers you that you are not fully protecting yourself."
Amplified reflection	Use when only the negative side of ambivalence is expressed; exaggerate or intensify what was said to lead the adolescent to correct the distortion. Use a light touch so that the comments are not heard as sarcastic or condescending (only works when there is some ambivalence about the behavior or situation).	Adolescent: "I only have sex with one person, so I know I won't get an STD." Clinician: "You really trust your partner and feel completely safe putting your life in his/her hands."

Agenda Setting

When the adolescent and health care provider can identify more than 1 sexual or contraceptive health behavior that could benefit from change (eg, enhancing pregnancy prevention for an adolescent who relies solely on condoms; enhancing STD prevention for an adolescent who uses a hormonal method but no condoms; discussing multiple options for an adolescent who is unsure if he or she wants to become sexually active or remain abstinent), setting an agenda can efficiently prioritize and focus discussion on 1 or 2 behaviors that the adolescent is most interested in and agrees to target. The goal of agenda setting is to understand the adolescent's agenda and let him or her select the behavior(s) to discuss. Individuals are more likely to change behaviors when they select the focus. The aim of the activity is to encourage the adolescent to decide what to talk about, with the assistance of the health care provider. In the realm of sexual and contraceptive behaviors, specific agenda-setting charts can be created to open up discussion on the range of different contraceptive options available. It can be helpful to write on the chart (see Fig 1) or, even better, to ask the adolescent to fill in the circles or to cross out items. The agenda-setting chart should not be used as a checklist or to create a premature focus on 1 behavior at the expense of others.

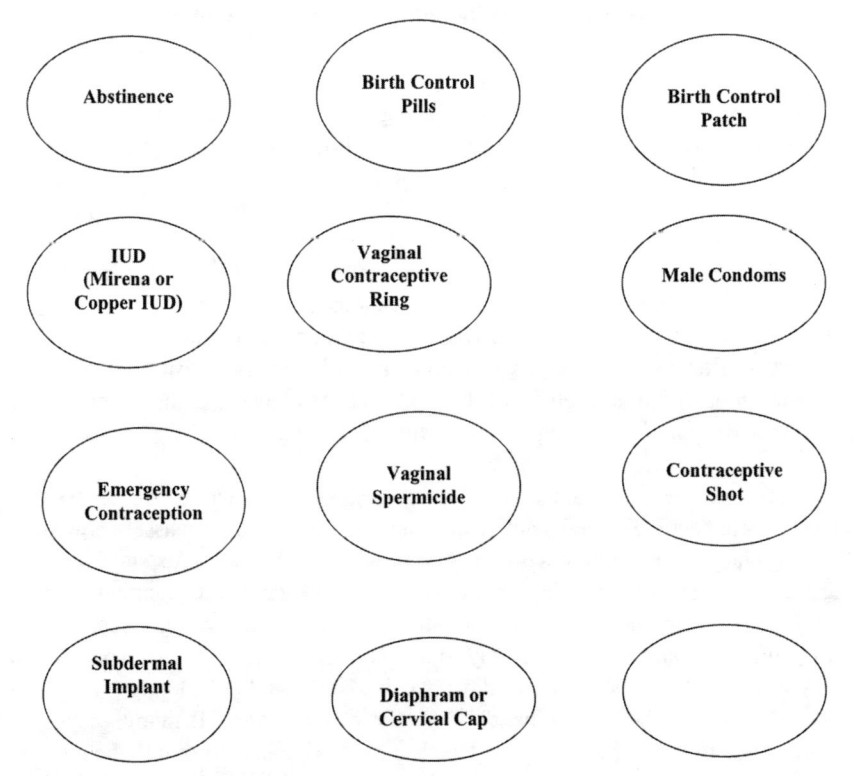

Fig 1. Agenda-setting chart.

The chart should be used to introduce the concept that the adolescent may be more ready to change 1 behavior over another. The adolescent will decide what he or she wishes to discuss.

Here is an example of how to introduce a contraceptive agenda-setting chart (see Fig 1): "On this chart are some things that help prevent pregnancy, STDs, and sometimes both. We could talk about abstinence, condoms, pills, the patch, the ring, IUDs, or emergency contraception, all of which can help you avoid pregnancy, and some can help you avoid STDs. You will be the best judge of what to consider using. Which of these do you think we could talk about today? This blank circle here is for anything else that you think might be of greater concern to you today. What should be in this space? What do you think? Which of these would you like to talk about today?"

CASES

The following cases provide examples of encounters with adolescents who are facing different sexual or contraceptive situations. Each case provides practical MI strategies and phrases that clinicians might choose to use in similar scenarios.

Case 1: Assessing Readiness to Remain Abstinent or Have Sex

> Brittany is a 15-year-old high school sophomore who comes to your office for a routine health visit. During the psychosocial history, Brittany tells you that she has been dating her boyfriend John for 6 months now, and they have been talking about having sex. Until now, they have only kissed. Brittany says that she is "the last of her friends to have sex," and she wants to start birth control "just in case." She is actively involved in her student government, the soccer team, and her local church's youth ministry. Brittany tells you that after graduating high school she plans to go to college to study to be an elementary school teacher. Brittany is unaccompanied for today's visit and says her mother would prefer that she wait longer to have sex; she is aware that Brittany is thinking about starting birth control.

Brittany may be ambivalent about becoming sexually active. To assess her readiness to become sexually active or remain abstinent, you can assess how soon she is planning to start having sex or how long she plans to stay sexually abstinent by asking specific questions: "How soon are you planning to start having sex? In the next few days, in a month or two, or are you not sure? When do you plan to start?" Another way to ask is to say, "How long do you plan to stay abstinent? For the next few days, weeks, or a couple of months? When do you plan to stop being abstinent?" Another way to assess Brittany's stage of readiness is to use a readiness ruler (see Fig 2). Asking her to point to the number that represents how she feels about change on a visual scale that shows the

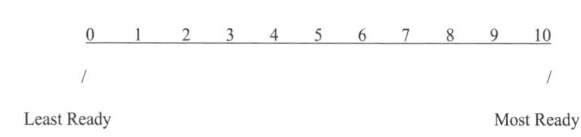

```
0   1   2   3   4   5   6   7   8   9   10
/                                        /
      Least Ready              Most Ready
```
Fig 2. Readiness ruler.

highest and lowest readiness levels can facilitate a discussion about decision-making. Exploring readiness can help resolve ambivalence and enhance motivation for change by incorporating the teen's own values and goals.

You could use a readiness ruler to assess Brittany's readiness to become sexually active by saying, "Brittany, I understand you are considering the decision about whether to become sexually active with John. Sometimes it helps to talk about where you are in terms of this decision, because you know what is right for you right now and how ready you are to make any changes. I'm going to ask you to look at this readiness ruler and tell me on a scale from 0 to 10, where 10 is the most ready and 0 is the least, how ready are you right now to start having sex?"

Depending on how Brittany responds will determine your next strategy. If she says, "Right now, I guess I'm about a 3," you would respond differently than if she says, "Right now, I am pretty ready. I would say I am an 8."

Once you obtain a readiness rating, the number will determine if you should focus on exploring the pros and cons of the current behavior (the status quo) or the pros and cons of change. If readiness to change is low (rated as a 0–5), explore all the perceived "good things" about the current behavior first by saying, "Brittany, it sounds like you are not completely ready right now to start having sex. Tell me what you like about being abstinent." Some helpful questions might include, "For you, what are the good things about being abstinent? What feels right about being abstinent? How does being abstinent fit with your goals and values? What makes you want to continue being abstinent?"

Keep asking Brittany what she likes about being abstinent or the good things about it until she says, "That's it" or "I can't think of any more." Summarize what she has said so far by saying, "So the good things for you about staying abstinent right now are __." Then, ask her to explore the other side or the "not-so-good things" about staying abstinent by saying, "Okay, so I hear that there are certain things that you really like, enjoy, and value about being abstinent [depending on what she said]. So, what is the other side? What are the not-so-good things about staying abstinent right now? What doesn't feel right about remaining abstinent right now? What is it that you don't like about it?" Keep asking Brittany what she does not like about being abstinent until she says, "That's it." Then, restate both sides of the decisional balance, presenting the not-so-good things about abstinence first, followed by the good things about it, and then ask, "So what do you want to do from here? Would it make more sense to start birth control right now, work on ways to stay abstinent, or something else? What do you think? What makes the most sense to you right now?"

If readiness to become sexually active is high, (rated as a 6–10) use this same dialogue to explore all the perceived good things of starting to have sex by saying, "You said your readiness is an 8. It sounds like you are really feeling ready to start having sex. So for you, what would be the good things right now about becoming sexually active?" Other helpful questions might include, "What do you like about the idea of having sex? What feels right about having sex? How does having sex fit with your goals and values? How does having sex fit with how you see your relationship with John? What makes you feel that now is the right time to start having sex?"

Keep asking Brittany what she sees as the good things about becoming sexually active until she says, "That's it." Respond by saying, "So the good things for you about having sex right now are __." Then, ask her to explore the other side or the not-so-good things about becoming sexually active by saying, "Okay, so I hear that there are certain things that you really like, enjoy, and value about having sex [depending on what she said]. So, what is the other side? What are the not-so-good things about becoming sexually active right now? What does not feel right about having sex? What is it that you don't like or worry about?" Keep asking Brittany what she does not like about becoming sexually active until she says, "That's it." Then, restate both sides of the decisional balance, presenting the good things about becoming sexually active first followed by the not-so-good things about it and then ask, "So what do you want to do from here? Would it make more sense to start birth control right now, work on ways to stay abstinent, something else? What do you think? What makes the most sense to you right now?"

Case 2: Importance and Confidence

> James is a 17-year-old young man who comes to your office complaining of a 2-day history of burning with urination. In obtaining the psychosocial history, James tells you that he had sex with a new partner last weekend, and he thinks "she has something." James states that he has had 3 lifetime partners, and he uses condoms "sometimes." He has no previous history of STDs. The rest of his history and his physical examination are normal. His urine test results are positive for moderate leukocytes. You tell James that you will send his urine for additional testing for specific infections but you think he has an STD; you offer him a prescription for the appropriate antibiotics.

You want to talk with James about his condom use; you want him to use them more consistently, if not every time he has sex, but you do not know yet how he feels about it. You could use the same readiness ruler as described in case 1 with Brittany to assess his readiness to use condoms more consistently (see Fig 2).

```
0    1    2    3    4    5    6    7    8    9    10
/                                                    /
Least Important                          Most Important


0    1    2    3    4    5    6    7    8    9    10
/                                                    /
Least Confident                          Most Confident
```
Fig 3. Example of importance and confidence rulers.

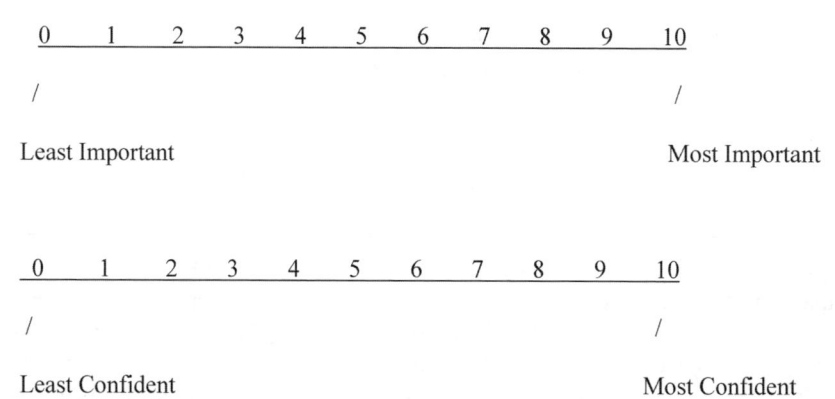

Another strategy might be to assess his perceived importance of and confidence in using condoms more often by saying, "James, given this recent infection, I would like to know how you feel right now about using condoms more often. It is up to you to decide what is best for you. I have 2 questions for you using these 2 rulers [see Fig 3]. First, how important is it to you to use condoms? Point to your importance level on this importance ruler, where 10 is the most important and 0 is the least important. How important is it to you right now to use condoms every time you have sex?" Wait for his response and then say, "Okay, here is the second question: If it was really important to you, how confident or sure are you that you could use condoms every time you have sex? Point to your confidence level on this confidence ruler, where 10 is the most confident and 0 is the least confident. How confident are you that you could use condoms every time you have sex if it was important to you?" Wait for his response.

The focus of your conversation with James will depend on how he rates importance and confidence. If 1 number is distinctly lower than the other, focus on the lower number first. If importance is low (≤ 5) or if both importance and confidence levels are nearly the same, focus on importance. If both are very low (≤ 3), explore his feelings about talking about using condoms in general.

For example, if James says that importance is a 3 and confidence is an 8, focus on importance, and ask, "What made you choose a 3 and not a lower number like a 1 or a 2? What makes using condoms this important?" Reflect the reasons given and ask for elaboration: "Tell me more about that." Then, ask for more reasons by saying, "What else makes it important?" Keep asking for reasons why importance is a 3 and not lower until he says, "That's it." Then, summarize what James said by saying, "So what makes this important right now is __." Do not allow him to tell you why the number is a 3 and not a higher number. You want him to talk about his reasons for using condoms, not the barriers against using them. Then ask, "What would have to happen to make using condoms a little bit more important to you?" Reflect and ask for elaboration by saying, "What else?" and reflecting until he says, "That's it." Then, summarize by saying, "So what makes using condoms important is __, and using condoms would be even more important if __." End the conversation with an open-ended question such as, "So what do you think you are going to do about using condoms in the future?"

If James says that importance is a 7 but his confidence is a 4, focus on confidence, and ask, "What made you choose a 4 and not a lower number like a 1 or a 2? What makes you feel confident that you can use condoms more often?" Reflect reasons given and ask for elaboration: "Tell me more about that." Then, ask for more reasons by saying, "What else makes you feel confident?" Keep asking for reasons why confidence is a 4 and not lower until he says, "That's it." Then, summarize what James said by saying, "So what makes you confident or sure that you can use condoms more right now is __." Do not allow him to tell you why the number is a 4 and not higher. You want him to talk about why he is confident that he can use condoms more often, not why he is not confident. Then ask, "What would have to happen for you to feel a little bit more confident that you could use condoms more often?" Reflect and ask for elaboration by saying, "What else?" Reflect until he says, "That's it." Then, summarize by saying, "So what makes you confident that you can use condoms more often is __, and you would feel more confident about using condoms if __." End the conversation with an open-ended question such as, "So what do you think you are going to do about using condoms in the future?" Note that this strategy, using importance and confidence rulers, could also have been used in case 1 with Brittany to assess how important it is for her to stay abstinent and how confident she is that she can stay abstinent if she wanted to do so.

Case 3: FRAMES Paragraph

> Jessica is a 19-year-old who presents to your office for a pregnancy test. She thinks she could be pregnant and says that she stopped taking her birth control pills 3 or 4 months ago because she could not remember to take them. She reports that her period is ~10 days late, and she had unprotected sex after her last menstrual period 2 weeks ago with her partner of 2 years. Her physical examination is unremarkable. She says that she has been thinking that she wants to be pregnant but she wonders if this is the right time. She smokes 1 pack of cigarettes per day and drinks 3 to 4 glasses of wine daily. Her urine pregnancy test results are negative.

The acronym FRAMES represents the 6 components of effective brief intervention: feedback, responsibility, advice, menu of options, empathy, and supporting self-efficacy.[18] One way to use these 6 components is to create a FRAMES paragraph that incorporates the history, physical, and laboratory findings into your interaction with Jessica. Below is an example of a FRAMES paragraph tailored to Jessica's case.

Feedback: Assessment of Current Status

"Jessica, your urine pregnancy test result is negative. Because the last time you had unprotected sex was 2 weeks ago, this is an accurate test. You said you smoke and drink alcohol daily. You also said you are thinking about getting pregnant and at the same time are not sure if now is the right time."

Responsibility: Emphasize Personal Choice

"It's up to you to decide when, or if, you are ready to have a baby. Only you can decide when the time is right."

Advice: Recommend Behavior Change

"Is it okay if I share with you what I think you should do right now?" Wait for affirmation and, if received, say, "The best thing you could do right now to have a healthy baby when you are ready is to not get pregnant until you stop smoking cigarettes and drinking alcohol and start taking folic acid so that when you do get pregnant, your baby will be healthy. What do you think of that suggestion?"

Menu of Options: Alternative Strategies or Options

"There are lots of ways you can avoid getting pregnant until you are ready. You could figure out a better way to remember the pills or switch to another method that might be easier to remember like the patch, the vaginal ring, or the shot, or perhaps there is something else you would rather do. What are some ideas you have about ways you could delay getting pregnant until you are ready?"

Empathy

"I know that making a decision about when to have a baby can be hard. It may seem like there is never a right time or that any time is fine."

Self-efficacy: Reinforce Hope and Optimism

"Let's look at your past successes to see what you learned from those experiences, and we can see how you could apply what you learned to this situation. I'm here to help you have a healthy pregnancy when you decide the time is right."

Case 4: Exchanging Information About Contraceptive Methods (Elicit-Provide-Elicit or Ask-Tell-Ask)

> Stephanie is a 16-year-old girl who comes to your office requesting emergency contraception because "the condom broke yesterday." She also mentions that she wants something "more reliable" for contracep-

tion. Some of her friends are on the pill, but she's not sure she'd be able to remember taking something every day. Her history, family history, and physical examination are unremarkable. Stephanie has had 1 previous sex partner. She reports that she had a "pregnancy scare" with her last partner because they did not use a condom every time.

A time-saving approach that helps provide information or advice when an adolescent may already have information or knowledge about a topic and can identify possible options for change is elicit-provide-elicit (also called "ask-tell-ask"). This approach can allow the health care provider to focus more on assisting the adolescent in making a plan that is realistic and successful rather than spending time providing unneeded information or advice. When information is missing or inaccurate after it is elicited from the adolescent, the provider may want to provide information. Before information is provided, the provider should always ask permission to give advice or information. Most importantly, after providing information, it is critical to elicit the adolescent's reaction to the information or advice that was given. The following is an example of how you might use elicit-provide-elicit with Stephanie.

Emphasize Personal Choice and Control

"Stephanie, what you decide to do about this is up to you. I can tell you about what works for other people, but you will be the best judge of what works for you."

Elicit Existing Knowledge/Experience

"Tell me what you know about your birth control options? What method do you think would work best for you and why? What have you heard about other methods that do not require daily use, such as Depo-Provera, the patch, and the vaginal ring? Summarize what she already knows and affirm her current knowledge by saying, "You really know a lot about this. It seems like you have been reading and talking with people and really care about your body and your health" Ask for elaboration of previous attempts/strategies by asking, "What methods have you used before? How well did they work for you? What happened when you tried using spermicide?"

Ask Permission

"Would it be okay if I told you more about the patch? There are some things others have found helpful for remembering to take the pill everyday. Would you be interested in hearing about them?" Affirm her interest/willingness. "I appreciate you being so open to new ideas and information."

Provide Information/Recommendations

"One thing that I have seen help other people remember to take their pills every day is to take it every morning when they brush their teeth or pair taking it with something they do already every day." Or, "Many people use their cell-phone alarm to remind themselves when to change their patch, take their pill, or get their shot." Use ordinary language, limit the quantity of information, and link it to identified goals. "How does getting the shot and waiting to have a baby until you are 25 years old fit with your future goals to be a television producer?"

Elicit Reactions/Interpretations

"What do you make of this? How do you feel about what we have been talking about? Which of the options I described seems like the best fit for you? What are your thoughts about trying the ring?" Reflect, and ask for elaboration: "What makes you think the patch would work for you? What is it about the ring that seems like it is the best choice for you right now?"

CONCLUSIONS

Clinicians who care for adolescents face many challenges when they encounter young people with sexual health–related issues. It can be especially challenging, because clinicians often have their own agendas. Many clinicians want adolescents to either stay abstinent or to always use condoms plus a hormonal contraceptive when they choose to be sexually active. Clinicians may want to tell adolescents, "Don't have sex!" "Always use condoms!" or "Get a Depo-Provera shot!" and know that it will result in behavior change. Clinicians might also be overly optimistic that their advice alone will result in health-related changes. Clinicians who are able to meet adolescents' readiness stage and work collaboratively to help them make change may have improved therapeutic interactions. More importantly, this connection will result in better outcomes. Clinicians facilitate adolescents' autonomy when they apply MI to sexual and contraceptive counseling. MI techniques also help clinicians offer information, advice, or skills that adolescents will be more likely to embrace and apply to many behavioral issues and future life situations. It is most important for clinicians to maintain the spirit of MI by eliciting from adolescents their perspectives and collaborating with them to share ideas, knowledge, and suggestions for behavior change. Good negotiation about sexual and contraceptive behavior change involves careful listening and strategic guiding by clinicians to support each adolescent's autonomy in making healthy choices.

REFERENCES

1. Petersen R, Payne P, Albright J, Holland H, Cabral R, Curtis KM. Applying motivational interviewing to contraceptive counseling: ESP for clinicians. *Contraception*. 2004;69(3):213–217
2. Rigotti NA, Park ER, Regan S, et al. Efficacy of telephone counseling for pregnant smokers: a randomized controlled trial. *Obstet Gynecol*. 2006;108(1):83–92
3. Thyrian JR, Hannöver W, Grempler J, Röske K, John U, Hapke U. An intervention to support postpartum women to quit smoking or remain smoke-free. *J Midwifery Womens Health*. 2006; 51(1):45–50

4. Suplee PD. The importance of providing smoking relapse counseling during the postpartum hospitalization. *J Obstet Gynecol Neonatal Nurs.* 2005;34(6):703–712
5. Tappin DM, Lumsden MA, Gilmour WH, et al. Randomised controlled trial of home based motivational interviewing by midwives to help pregnant smokers quit or cut down. *BMJ.* 2005;331(7513):373–377
6. Stotts AL, DeLaune KA, Schmitz JM, Grabowski J. Impact of a motivational intervention on mechanisms of change in low-income pregnant smokers. *Addict Behav.* 2004;29(8):1649–1657
7. Stotts AL, DiClemente CC, Dolan-Mullen P. One-to-one: a motivational intervention for resistant pregnant smokers. *Addict Behav.* 2002;27(2):275–292
8. Valanis B, Lichtenstein E, Mullooly JP, et al. Maternal smoking cessation and relapse prevention during health care visits. *Am J Prev Med.* 2001;20(1):1–8
9. Tappin DM, Lumsden MA, McIntyre D, et al. A pilot study to establish a randomized trial methodology to test the efficacy of a behavioural intervention. *Health Educ Res.* 2000;15(4): 491–502
10. Velasquez MM, Hecht J, Quinn VP, Emmons KM, DiClemente CC, Dolan-Mullen P. Application of motivational interviewing to prenatal smoking cessation: training and implementation issues. *Tob Control.* 2000;9(suppl 3):III36-III40
11. Handmaker NS, Wilbourne P. Motivational interventions in prenatal clinics. *Alcohol Res Health.* 2001;25(3):219-21-9
12. Handmaker NS, Miller WR, Manicke M. Findings of a pilot study of motivational interviewing with pregnant drinkers. *J Stud Alcohol.* 1999;60(2):285–287
13. Handmaker NS, Hester RK, Delaney HD. Videotaped training in alcohol counseling for obstetric care practitioners: a randomized controlled trial. *Obstet Gynecol.* 1999;93(2):213–218
14. Ingersoll K, Floyd L, Sobell M, Velasquez MM; Project CHOICES Intervention Research Group. Reducing the risk of alcohol-exposed pregnancies: a study of a motivational intervention in community settings. *Pediatrics.* 2003;111(5 pt 2):1131–1135
15. Ingersoll KS, Ceperich SD, Nettleman MD, Karanda K, Brocksen S, Johnson BA. Reducing alcohol-exposed pregnancy risk in college women: initial outcomes of a clinical trial of a motivational intervention. *J Subst Abuse Treat.* 2005;29(3):173–180
16. Ott MA, Labbett RL, Gold MA. Counseling adolescents about abstinence in the office setting. *J Pediatr Adolesc Gynecol.* 2007;20(1):39–44
17. Conard LE, Gold MA. Emergency contraception update: providing emergency contraception in the pediatrician's office. *Contemp Pediatr.* 2006;23(2):49–70
18. Bien TH, Miller WR, Tonigan JS. Brief interventions for alcohol problems: a review. *Addiction.* 1993;88(3):315–336

RESOURCES

Gold MA. Case commentary: gynecological care for adolescents. *Virtual Mentor.* 2003;5(5). Available at: http://virtualmentor.ama-assn.org/2003/05/ccas1-0305.html. Accessed May 2, 2003 [case commentary that illustrates the use of the transtheoretical model and motivational interviewing style into practical approaches to providing reproductive health care to a female adolescent]

Miller WR, Rollnick S. *Motivational Interviewing: Preparing People for Change.* 2nd ed. New York, NY: Guilford Press; 2002 [the essential textbook on motivational interviewing]

Rollnick S, Mason P, Butler C. *Health Behavior Change: A Guide for Practitioners.* London, United Kingdom: Churchill Livingstone; 199 [a paperback (good value) recommended for those interested in further expanding their knowledge of motivational interviewing in the health care setting including behavior change counseling]

Dunn C, Rollnick S. *Lifestyle Change.* Philadelphia, PA: Mosby/Elsevier Ltd; 2003 [small pocket-sized paperback book; part of the Rapid Reference Series, which focuses on motivational interviewing in the medical setting]

Helping Adolescents to Stop Using Drugs: Role of the Primary Care Clinician

Sharon Levy, MD, MPH[a,b,c,d]*, John R. Knight, MD[a,b,c,d,e,f]

[a]Department of Pediatrics, Harvard Medical School, 25 Shattuck Street, Boston, MA 02115, USA

[b]Center for Adolescent Substance Abuse Research, [c]Division of Developmental Medicine, [d]Department of Psychiatry, Children's Hospital Boston, 300 Longwood Avenue, Boston, MA 02115

[e]Division on Addictions, Harvard Medical School, 25 Shattuck Street, Boston, MA 02115, USA

[f]Division of Adolescent/Young Adult Medicine, Children's Hospital Boston, 300 Longwood Avenue, Boston, MA 02115, USA

Substance use is common during adolescence and has significant long- and short-term health consequences. Primary care clinicians are in the ideal situation to detect substance use, and the *Bright Futures* guidelines recommend screening all adolescents for alcohol and other drug use at each yearly health maintenance visit.[1] In this article we describe methods for screening, assessment, and very brief interventions that can be performed within a primary care visit. We use case scenarios to demonstrate the use of theoretical models within the course of a primary care encounter to briefly assess an adolescent with a positive screening-test result for a substance use disorder and determine his or her readiness to change. With this information, a primary care clinician can use principles of motivational interviewing (MI) to create a very brief intervention that challenges the teen to make a change or prepares them to accept a referral for treatment.

All adolescents should be screened for drug and alcohol use at every primary care encounter. We recommend beginning the discussion with 3 questions regarding the use of drugs and alcohol (see Table 1). If all 3 of these questions are answered "no," the clinician should give positive reinforcement before moving on to the next portion of the history. If any of these questions are answered "yes," the clinician should administer a screening test, such as the CRAFFT questions,[2] to determine level of risk. CRAFFT is a mnemonic acronym created from the first letters of key words in the test's 6 questions (car, relax, alone, forget, friends, trouble), as described in Table 1.

---

*Corresponding author.
E-mail address: Sharon.Levy@childrens.harvard.edu (S. Levy).

Copyright © 2008 American Academy of Pediatrics. All rights reserved. ISSN 1934-4287

Table 1
Opening questions about drug and alcohol use and the CRAFFT questions

Initial questions
    "Have you ever drank alcohol (more than a few sips)?"
    "Have you ever used marijuana or hashish?"
    "Have you ever used any other drug to get high? By 'other drug' we mean illicit drugs (such as ecstasy or heroin), prescription drugs such as OxyContin or Klonopin that were not prescribed by your doctor or taken the way the doctor said to, over-the-counter medications (such as dextromethorphan), and inhalants such as glue or nitrous from spray cans."
CRAFFT questions: during the past 12 mo
    "Have you ever ridden in a car driven by someone (including yourself) who was 'high' or had been using alcohol or drugs?"
    "Do you ever use alcohol or drugs to relax, feel better about yourself, or fit in?"
    "Do you ever use alcohol or drugs while you are by yourself, alone?"
    "Do you ever forget things you did while using alcohol or drugs?"
    "Do your family or friends ever tell you that you should cut down on your drinking or drug use?"
    "Have you ever gotten into trouble while you were using alcohol or drugs?"

Table 2
Sample brief advice

Health effects of substance use
    "Drugs and alcohol affect your brain and can damage it for life."
    "Alcohol can hurt your liver."
    "Smoked drugs, including marijuana, can hurt your lungs"
    "Smoking marijuana increases your risk of developing depression and schizophrenia (psychosis)."
    "Alcohol and drugs, including marijuana, impair driving ability and can cause accidents."
    "Drug and alcohol use puts teens at higher risk of sexual assault, sexually transmitted infections, and unwanted pregnancy."
    "If a girl becomes pregnant, drug and alcohol use can hurt the baby."
Driving/riding while intoxicated:
    "Drug- and alcohol-related car crashes are a leading cause of death for young people."
    "Don't ever drive a car after using drugs or drinking, even if you don't feel 'high' or drunk."
    "Make arrangements ahead of time for safe transportation."
    "Please talk to your parents about the 'contract for life.' I'd like you to come back in a week and let me know how that conversation went"

Each "yes" response is scored 1 point. A score of ≥2 is a positive screen result and indicates that the adolescent is at high risk for having an alcohol- or drug-related disorder and in need of further assessment. Patients who have used alcohol or another drug but have a CRAFFT score of 0 or 1 may benefit from brief advice regarding the negative health effects of the substance they are using. Clinicians should use their knowledge of the patient to personalize the advice statement as much as possible. Brief advice can be given quickly and may make an impact on teens with low-risk substance use. Table 2 provides examples of brief advice statements.

In this article we present strategies that can be used to engage adolescents in discussing substance use when a CRAFFT screen result is positive. We begin with 2 theoretical models: "stages of use,"[3] which describes the spectrum of drug use from experimentation to substance dependence, and "stages of change," which was developed by Prochaska and DiClemente[4] and maps out the incremental cognitive steps necessary for behavioral change to occur. In the next section we discuss adolescents who use alcohol and marijuana, because the high cultural acceptability of these drugs can lead to minimization and underrecognition of disorders with these substances. We then discuss misuse of over-the-counter and prescription medication, which is on the rise nationally, and use of other illegal drugs.

THEORETICAL MODELS

Stages of Use

The use of substances forms a spectrum, with each stage representing a different relationship between the adolescent and the substance. Although the time spent in each stage may vary among individuals and specific substances, the stages are most often passed through in the same order of progression.

The essence of each stage of use is described in Table 3.

The stage of use is typically underestimated by adolescents and frequently by parents as well. Alcohol and drug use is often referred to as "experimental" because of an adolescent's age, without regard to level of previous experience, motives, or associated problems. In some clinical instances, discussing a teenager's current stage of use and the implications can provide both a motivation to change for the adolescent as well as a realistic assessment for the parents.

Stages of Change

The stages-of-change model delineates the steps through which an individual passes in the process of changing a behavior. As with the stages of use, the amount of time spent in any 1 stage will vary among individuals, but the stages are usually passed through in the same order. Table 4 defines each of the stages of behavioral change.

The stages of use and stages of change are roughly correlated but do not overlap entirely, and in many cases patients' perceived stage of use may be more predictive of their stage of change than their actual stage of use. Understanding where an adolescent fits on these 2 models can help the clinician set intervention goals and determine the most appropriate strategy for working with the adolescent. Graphic representations of these models, such as those shown in Figs 1 and 2, may be helpful teaching tools. The clinician can begin by describing each of

Table 3
Stages of use

Stage	Description
Abstinence	The time before a teenager has ever tried drugs or more than a few sips of alcohol
Experimentation	The first 1 or 2 times that a substance is used; experimentation is generally of shorter duration; an adolescent who is experimenting is curious to know what it feels like to be intoxicated
Regular (nonproblematic) use	Drug use together with 1 or more friends for recreational purposes in relatively low-risk situations and without related problems; regular use typically occurs at predictable times such as on weekends
Problematic use	Drug use in a high-risk situation (such as in a car or when baby-sitting), associated with a problem (such as a fight while intoxicated, a school suspension or arrest), or for purposes other than recreation (such as to relieve stress or depression)
Substance abuse	Continued substance use despite a significant negative impact on functioning as defined in the fourth edition of the DSM-IV[8]
	A maladaptive pattern of substance use that leads to clinically significant impairment or distress as manifested by 1 (or more) of the following, occurring within a 12-mo period
	Recurrent substance use that results in a failure to fulfill major role obligations at work, school, or home
	Recurrent substance use in situations in which it is physically hazardous
	Recurrent substance-related legal problems
	Continued use despite having persistent or recurrent social or interpersonal problems caused or exacerbated by the effects of the substance
Substance dependence	Loss of control over use of a substance, or compulsion to use a substance, as defined in the DSM-IV
	A maladaptive pattern of substance use that leads to clinically significant impairment or distress, as manifested by 3 or more of the following, occurring any time in the same 12-mo period
	Tolerance
	Withdrawal
	The substance is often taken in larger amounts or over a longer period than intended
	There is a persistent desire or unsuccessful efforts to cut down or control substance use
	A great deal of time is spent in activities necessary to obtain the substance, use the substance, or recover from its effects
	Important social, occupational, or recreational activities are given up or reduced because of substance use
	The substance use is continued despite knowledge of having a persistent physical or psychological problem that is likely to have been caused or exacerbated by the substance

DSM-IV indicates the fourth edition of the Diagnostic and Statistical Manual of Mental Disorders.

Table 4
Stages of change

Stage	Description
Precontemplation	The adolescent does not believe that his or her substance use has or will cause problems and has not begun to consider a change.
Contemplation	The adolescent begins to consider the negative impact of substance use and weighs the reasons to continue against the reasons to stop.
Determination	The adolescent has decided to make a change, but no action has occurred yet. This stage may involve setting a quit date or agreeing to see a counselor.
Action	The adolescent has made a behavioral change.
Maintenance	The behavior change has been well established. The adolescent may continue to develop new strategies to avoid substance use in a variety of settings.
Relapse	A recurrence of substance use after achieving abstinence. A single use or use over a brief period of time with a quick return to commitment to abstinence is often referred to as a "slip." This is in distinction to a loss of commitment to change, which is referred to as a relapse.

the stages and then asking the patient how his or her use would best be described. Once a patient understands the description of each stage, he or she may reinterpret his or her own level of use. Table 5 lists strategies that are appropriate for using at various stages of use and stages of change.

ADOLESCENT DRUG AND ALCOHOL USE: A DEVELOPMENTAL VIEW

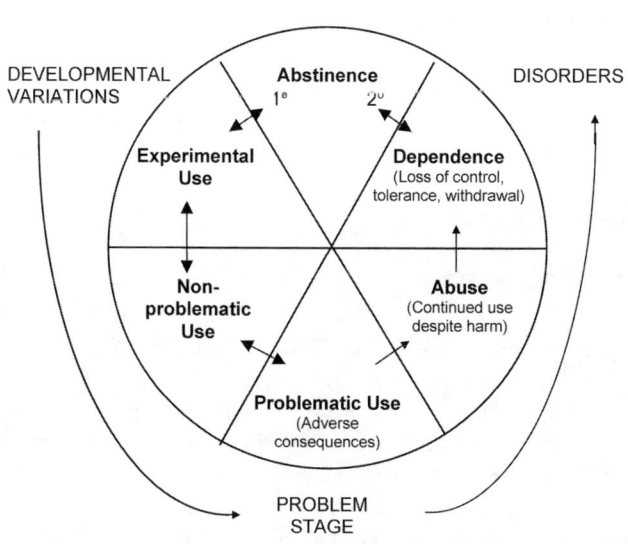

Fig 1. Adolescent drug and alcohol use: a developmental view. 1° indicates primary. 2° indicates secondary. Sources: Knight JR. *Contemp Pediatr.* 1997:14(4):45–72; and Wolraich ML, ed. *The Classification of Child and Adolescent Mental Diagnoses in Primary Care.* Elk Grove Village, IL: American Academy of Pediatrics; 1996.

(Prochaska and DiClemente)

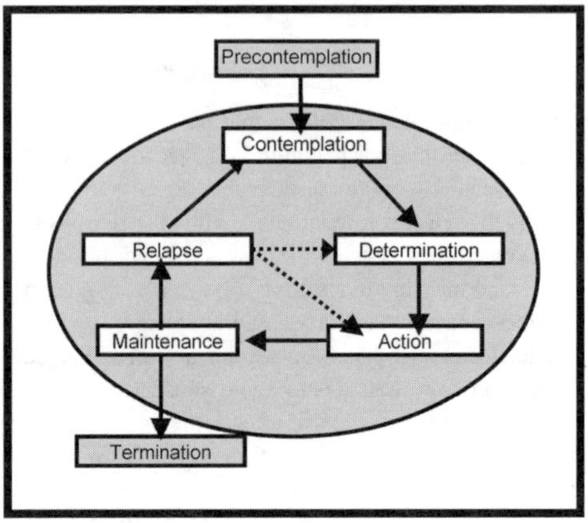

Fig 2. Stages of change. Sources: Prochaska JO, Velicer WF, Rossi JS, et al. *Health Psychol.* 1994;13(1):39–46; and Prochaska JO. *Health Psychol.* 1994;13(1):47–51.

MOTIVATIONAL INTERVIEWING

The strategies presented in Table 2 are based on the principles of MI,[5] which are reviewed in depth by another article in this issue.[6] Briefly, MI is a style of interpersonal interactions that creates conditions that are favorable for behavior change. MI is based on the assumption that motivation and ambivalence are not innate character traits but, rather, situational states. Four basic principles guide MI: (1) the clinician strives to help the adolescent develop a discrepancy between current behaviors and future goals; (2) when an adolescent becomes resistant, the clinician should find common ground and change the direction of the conversation; (3) the clinician should always encourage and support the patient's sense of self-efficacy; and (4) the clinician should always be empathetic to create the conditions necessary for change.

CASE VIGNETTES

Alcohol and Marijuana

> A 16-year-old girl tells you that she drinks 2 to 3 times per month on weekends at parties with friends. She is an "A" student, captain of the girls' basketball team, and volunteers several hours per week for a community-service organization. Her CRAFFT score is 2, and on further exploration she tells you that 1 month ago she had a blackout after drinking too much and does not know how she got home that night. Her parents know about that incident, and she gives you permission to discuss it with her mother after she joins you in the examination room. Her mother says that she understands that all adolescents drink from time to time, and she attributes the blackout to "inexperience and adolescent experimentation."

Table 5
Strategies appropriate for various stages of use and stages of change

Stage of Use	Stage of Change	Intervention Strategy	Intervention Goal
Abstinence	NA	Praise and encouragement	Indicate to the adolescent an openness to discussing drug and alcohol use in the future.
Experimentation or regular use	Precontemplation	Ask open-ended questions about the risks associated with drug use.	Raise concerns regarding continued drug use.
	Contemplation	Ask about the reasons for considering a behavior change. Provide valid medical information.	Draw out and further explore reasons for quitting.
Problem use or abuse	Precontemplation	Have the patient describe the problem associated with use. Listen reflectively by repeating the problem and any associated negative affect.	Consider the personal negative effects of drug use.
	Contemplation	Ask about problems associated with drug use and personal goals, and explore the discrepancy between those goals and current behavior. Weigh the pros and cons of continued use, and the pros and cons of behavioral change.	Agree to a trial of abstinence.
	Action	Ask about confidence in ability to sustain the change and previous motivations to use drugs. Develop strategies for avoiding drug use.	Maintain abstinence.
	Maintenance	Ask about risky situations and how drug use was avoided. Devise new strategies for avoiding use. Ask about pros and cons of abstinence.	Promote continued motivation to maintain abstinence.

(*Continued*)

Table 5
(*Continued*)

Stage of Use	Stage of Change	Intervention Strategy	Intervention Goal
	Relapse	Ask about the context of repeat drug use. Determine strength of commitment to abstinence. Develop new strategies for use in high-risk situations. Identify additional supports.	Return to abstinence.
Dependence	Contemplation	Determine the importance of change and confidence in ability to make a change. Support self-efficacy.	Agree to work toward change. Accept a referral to treatment.
	Action	Ask about barriers to change.	Identify appropriate level of services.
	Maintenance	Ask about the treatment, progress, and personal goals for the future.	Maintain therapeutic alliance.
	Relapse	Support self-efficacy. Reaffirm goals. Discuss the medical model of drug dependence and need for ongoing treatment.	Assist in getting back into treatment.

NA indicates not applicable.

This young woman had a serious risk associated with her drinking, and her stage of use would best be classified as problematic use. However, both the patient and her mother seem to have normalized her drinking and are describing her drinking pattern as "experimental"; her stage of change is precontemplation. In this circumstance, both the patient and her mother would likely reject the clinician's assessment of an alcohol problem at this point. An intervention may best begin by the clinician having the adolescent describe what she likes about drinking and then explore the circumstances of her blackout more thoroughly. The clinician can then summarize the pros and cons of drinking and ask the patient whether she would like to make a change to avoid the negative aspects of drinking in the future.

A 15-year-old boy tells you that he has been drinking approximately twice per month with friends for the past 6 months. He usually will have 5 to 6 beers over the course of the evening, which is enough to get him drunk. His CRAFFT score is 0. He often sleeps at a friend's house after drinking, and his parents do not know about his use of alcohol.

This young man is in the regular or nonproblematic stage of substance use, and he is likely in precontemplation. However, his young age places him at risk for acute problems associated with alcohol use and significantly increases his risk of developing a substance use disorder in the future.[7] He has been careful to hide his alcohol use from his parents by choosing to stay with a friend rather than come home and risk being caught drunk. A clinician could begin a conversation with open-ended questions regarding his parents. For example, "How would your parents feel if they knew that you were drinking? Why would they be so concerned?" Adolescents often project their own negative reasons for drinking onto their parents; giving this young man the opportunity to do so may move him from precontemplation into contemplation. The physician should challenge the young man to stop drinking for a very brief period of time: "Do you think you could stop drinking completely for a week or two? I would like to see if it is possible for you to do it. If you can, we can be reassured a bit that you haven't lost control. If you're unable to do it, for any reason, it may mean that you need to get help." The patient may not agree to this challenge; if this is the case, he may be willing to "think about it." In either case, he should be asked to come for a return visit to discuss his alcohol use further.

> A 17-year-old boy that you have known for several years presents for a health maintenance visit. He is doing well in school and is active in sports. He will graduate high school in the spring and has already been accepted to college. He has drank alcohol a few times in the past but does not like to be drunk, so he has not continued drinking. He uses marijuana intermittently, ~1 to 2 times per month; he does not consider his marijuana use a problem. He has never used other drugs. His CRAFFT score is 1 because he has ridden in a car with friends after smoking marijuana. When you ask him about that night he tells you that he knows that it is dangerous to ride with a driver who has been using marijuana but that sometimes that is the only practical way home.

This young man's use is best described as regular or nonproblematic, and he is in precontemplation. However, he has put himself at risk by riding with an intoxicated driver, and he is ambivalent about this risk. The clinician should explore this further by asking him why he thinks it is dangerous to ride with an intoxicated driver to emphasize his own understanding of the risk and then challenging him regarding how he might change things to avoid this risk with a statement such as, "So taking a ride home with your friends can be convenient, but you worry that you could end up in a car accident. What do you think you should do about that?" If the patient does not come up with solutions on his own, the clinician could ask for permission to share some strategies. For example, "Can I share with you some of the ideas I have heard from other kids? Some kids in the neighborhood have told me that they always carry an extra subway token in their pocket, or, if they are really stuck, sleep over at a friend's house. Would either of these strategies work for you? What else could you do?"

> An 18-year-old boy reports a 3-year history of marijuana use, smoking 1 to 2 times per week, on the weekends, with his friends. His CRAFFT score is 1; he reports that he has driven many times after smoking marijuana. He then adds that he believes that he is a much better driver after smoking marijuana, because he is "much more focused." However, he is not happy that he has gained 7 pounds since his last physical, which he attributes to having "the munchies" after smoking marijuana. He denies any other trouble associated with marijuana use and says that his parents do not know about his drug use.

This young man meets criteria for marijuana abuse, because he is recurrently putting himself in danger by driving while intoxicated. His stage of change is contemplation; he has volunteered that he believes he is a better driver when intoxicated, which suggests that he has spent some time thinking about the issue. He also attributes his weight gain, about which he is unhappy, to his substance use. Despite his contemplation, he has developed strong defenses in support of continuing to smoke marijuana, which are currently driving his behavior. Knowing that he is speaking with a physician who will not endorse his driving while intoxicated, he is likely expecting to be contradicted. It is important to begin an intervention with this patient by finding common ground. For example, the clinician could begin by telling the patient that many people believe that they are better drivers after smoking marijuana, and there are physiologic reasons for that belief. At this point, the clinician could then offer education on the effects of marijuana. For example, "We know that there are many types of focus. For example, the focus you need when you are performing a tedious task is very different from the type of focus you need for driving. Marijuana increases your focus on a single point. So after smoking, people may feel more focused, and in a way they are. But what do you think that kind of focus would do to your ability to drive? How else could you get around if you decided you did not want to drive after smoking?"

> A 15-year-old boy reports that he has been using marijuana 1 to 3 times per day for the past 6 months. His CRAFFT score is 5. He tells you that he primarily uses marijuana to relax and relieve stress. He describes escalating use of marijuana consistent with developing tolerance, and he tells you that he experienced withdrawal symptoms of headache and anxiety when he was away with his family for the weekend and could not smoke. He admits that he is usually high most of the day. His grades have fallen, although he attributes the decline to a general lack of interest in school and not to his marijuana use. He was arrested on 1 occasion when a police officer saw him smoking in a parked car, although he feels that he was particularly unlucky because several of his friends have been issued warnings in similar situations. He had thought about quitting a few months ago, because smoking makes it hard for him to play basketball, but he changed his mind

when he did not make the team. His smoking has created tension with his parents, who have punished him by taking away privileges on several occasions.

This young man has a diagnosis of cannabis dependence (he has demonstrated tolerance and withdrawal, spends a great deal of time under the influence of marijuana, and has failed to fulfill major role obligations at school) and has been thinking about quitting but remains ambivalent. Marijuana disorders can be particularly difficult to treat, because problems associated with marijuana use tend to be insidious and, as such, the causal relationship between problems and substance use may not be identified by the patient. (In this case, the young man does not associate his declining school performance with increasing marijuana use.) Many patients do not believe that marijuana is an addictive substance. Furthermore, patients with marijuana disorders often lack the motivation to produce the "activation energy" necessary for making and sustaining a behavior change.

A clinician could begin an intervention for this patient by exploring both his desire to change and his confidence that he would be able to sustain a change. One way to do this is by saying, "On a 10-point scale, where 10 is 'very much' and 1 is 'not at all,' where would you place your desire to stop stopping marijuana?" When he responds with "3," you then can say, "Tell me why you didn't pick '1' or '2.'" In this way you will elicit from him reasons to make a change. In a similar fashion, you can ask him to rank on a 10-point scale how confident he is in his ability to make a change if he wanted to, and ask why he did not choose a lower number to elicit from him his own strengths in quitting. It is likely that he is willing to consider a change in his marijuana use, because he has considered quitting before. The clinician must be careful to support that inclination while avoiding strengthening his reasons to continue smoking. Statements such as, "What's most important here is that you have previously decided to stop using marijuana" will remind him that making the change was his idea and his decision and may allow him to accept a referral for additional evaluation. Asking him about his motives for using marijuana can help to direct the types of supports he will need to be successful.

Prescription and Over-the-Counter Medications

> A 17-year-old girl tells you that she has used oxycodone to get high on 4 occasions. She uses it with her boyfriend and a new group of friends who are much more experienced than she is. Her CRAFFT score is 2; she has ridden with a driver who has smoked marijuana, and she has forgotten things that have happened after using oxycodone. She denies any trouble associated with drug use and tells you that she uses much less than her friends and is sure that she can control her use.

This young woman has a diagnosis of problematic use of opioids but is at high risk for quickly progressing to abuse and dependence because of the highly addictive nature of her substance of choice. She seems to be in precontemplation and a long way from being willing to make a behavioral change. She has not yet experienced serious negative consequences related to her drug use, but she has placed herself in a risky situation by being impaired enough to forget some of the things that happened to her when she was using oxycodone. The clinician could begin an intervention by asking her to describe the events around memory loss and asking her open-ended questions such as, "Have you considered what could have happened to you during that time you can't remember?" Her boyfriend and new group of drug-using friends are likely to have experienced many negative consequences associated with drug use, and she may be able to describe them. The clinician might also ask her to list warning signs of a drug problem and ask if she would include spending most of her time with friends who have drug problems.

Adolescents who present in precontemplation are usually not moved into action in the course of a single brief office intervention such as that described above. It is most practical to try to move your patient 1 stage of change forward during each office encounter. However, the intervention may be quite powerful if the adolescent continues to think about the questions posed during the next few days. Therefore, it is important with ambivalent patients to schedule a follow-up visit within 1 to 2 weeks. At the follow-up visit the clinician can simply ask the patient if she remembers what was discussed at the last meeting and whether she has thought about any of the questions. It also provides a good opportunity for the clinician to ask the patient whether she has any questions about the medical consequences of opioid or other drug use.

> A 14-year-old girl tells you that she uses stimulant medication alone in her room almost every weekend to help her study. Her CRAFFT score is 2; her best friend knows about her drug use and is worried about her. She is an "A" student and says she would not be able to do her work without the pills. She varies the dosage by how much she has to study, but lately she has been using more than she originally planned to use. She usually swallows the pills, but on 1 recent occasion she ground up the pills and insufflated them nasally to see if that would help her study even harder. She denies problems associated with drug use but worries that if she continues to use she will be caught by her parents or teachers. She tells you that she really wants to stop using, but does not know what else she can do to help her with her schoolwork.

This young woman's use is best described as problematic use, but she is at high risk of progressing quickly to abuse and dependence. She already likely has developed tolerance. She is in the stage of change of determination; she has made a decision to stop using drugs but has not yet changed her behavior. In this case, a clinician might begin an intervention by simply supporting her decision to stop using, acknowledging that it may be difficult at times, and assuring her that you will help her find support. Given her age, it would be best to work toward having her parents involved in further assessment and treatment. The clinician could start this conversation by saying, "It sounds as if you have decided that you want to stop taking stimulants but are not sure how to do that. I'd like to help you find support, and that would be easiest if your parents were able to help you with this. How do you think they would react if we told them that you had been using stimulants to help you study but that you decided that you want to stop and need their help?" The patient would benefit from a psychopharmacology evaluation to determine if she truly has attention-deficit/hyperactivity disorder, although many adolescents who misuse stimulants do not meet diagnostic criteria for this disorder. A referral for individual counseling and neuropsychological testing also may be helpful.

> A 16-year-old boy tells you that he has been using over-the-counter cough preparations that contain dextromethorphan to get high a few times each month for the past several months. His CRAFFT score is 4; he has driven with friends who have used drugs, he has used cough medicines alone in his room, he had forgotten what has happened after drinking a whole box of cough medicine on 1 occasion, and once he was in trouble after his parents found empty cough medicine boxes in his room (they suspended his allowance for 1 month). He told his parents that he stopped using drugs; his parents believed him, because results from a series of home drug tests were negative. One of his friends overdosed on cough medication and ended up in the emergency department, but he was discharged 12 hours later. The patient tells you that his "friend was stupid, but I know how to control myself." He says that he knows that he will stop using drugs at some point when he is older but does not see the need to stop now, because he does not have a problem.

This young man has problematic use of dextromethorphan and is currently in the contemplation stage of change. He has already decided that he will stop using drugs at some point. A clinician could begin an intervention by asking him what his goals are for the future. Once identified, one could then ask him how use of drugs would likely affect his goals–would it help him get closer, or push him further away? This conversation will elicit his ambivalence toward continued drug use. In this case, the clinician should also meet with the patient's parents and discuss alternatives to home drug testing, which will not detect dextromethorphan. Parents could monitor this young man by checking on his whereabouts after school and who he is with and also by checking his room on a regular basis to look for drugs, medication containers, or drug paraphernalia. Room searches should be performed with the teen's knowledge but without previous warning, and the parents should invite the teen to accompany them when they begin the search.

Other Drugs

> An 18-year-old girl tells you that she has a history of occasional drinking and marijuana use over the past year; more recently, she has used cocaine twice, each time at a night club with friends. Her CRAFFT score is 2. She used cocaine to "fit in" with her friends, and she once got in trouble for sneaking alcohol into a school dance. She does not report any trouble related to her use of cocaine. She says that many of her friends use cocaine once in a while and are not addicted; she does not think occasional use is a big deal.

Overall, this young woman's use of alcohol is best described as problematic, whereas her use of cocaine is experimental. Nonetheless, the phases of experimentation and regular use may be very short for a teenager who is experimenting with cocaine because of the highly addictive nature of the drug. In addition, her positive CRAFFT score suggests that she is at high risk of developing a drug or alcohol disorder. Her responses to the clinician's questions suggest that she is in the contemplation stage of change; she has thought about the risk of addiction to cocaine and has developed defensive responses. An intervention for her might best begin with open-ended questions such as, "What happens to people who do get addicted to cocaine?" or "How do people get addicted to cocaine? How would you know if you were developing a problem with cocaine?" The clinician might also ask her what she knows about the medical effects of cocaine and whether she has any questions about cocaine use.

CONFIDENTIALITY

Health care providers should ask questions regarding substance use in private after explaining the rules of confidentiality. Details recorded in the medical chart should be limited to information that supports or helps to rule out a diagnosis. Adolescents should be afforded confidentiality unless their behavior poses an acute safety risk to themselves or others. Determining whether a specific behavior presents a safety risk is a matter of clinical judgment; the patient's age, other diagnoses, and social situation should be taken into account. Occasional use of alcohol or marijuana can usually be kept confidential; drug binges or intravenous drug use usually indicate a need for treatment, about which parents must be informed.

Adolescents should be assured that when confidentiality must be broken, the health care provider and patient will review what will be said before speaking with the parents. Generally, the clinician should limit the disclosure to information specific to the acute risk, diagnostic information, and treatment recommendations. If the parents begin to ask the adolescent questions about specific details (ie, "Where did you get drugs? Who did you use drugs with?"), the clinician should be prepared to help redirect them. Although this information may ultimately be important during treatment, aggressive questioning at the time of the disclosure is likely to be difficult for the adolescent and may make him or her resistant to further assessment or entering treatment. Parents should understand that revealing too much information poses a risk to the therapeutic alliance between the provider and the young person.

CONCLUSIONS

Drug and alcohol use by adolescents can be detected by the use of simple screening questions. Many teenagers who have used alcohol and marijuana will be at low risk for a serious drug use problem and benefit from very brief advice from a clinician. Adolescents who have a positive CRAFFT score are at high risk for a substance use problem or disorder, and the clinician should gather additional history to determine both the stage of use and the stage of change. This information allows the clinician to have a brief yet meaningful therapeutic conversation.

The stages-of-change model predicts that successful interventions with adolescents in precontemplation or contemplation may not yield observable behavioral change right away. The goal of working with adolescents in these stages is to move them to consider behavioral change and to weigh the benefits and consequences of continuing their current behavior. In these cases, a follow-up appointment scheduled 1 to 2 weeks after the initial intervention is important. At the follow-up appointment the adolescent may be much more amenable to making a behavior change, and the clinician can help him or her move into the next stage of change or make a referral for additional services.

Some adolescents will not be ready to make a change or accept a treatment referral even after a skilled intervention. In these cases parents may be needed to help facilitate a referral to more structured treatment, and the clinician should consider whether breaking the adolescent's confidentiality is warranted, particularly if a substance use disorder is present. If the clinician decides to maintain the adolescent's confidentiality, the clinician should convey regard, concern, and availability: "I care about you, I am concerned about you, and I will be here for you."

REFERENCES

1. Green M, Palfrey J, eds. *Bright Futures: Guidelines for Health Supervision of Infants, Children, and Adolescents.* 2nd ed. Arlington, VA: National Center for Education in Maternal and Child Health; 2000
2. Knight JR, Sherritt L, Shrier LA, Harris SK, Chang G. Validity of the CRAFFT substance abuse screening test among adolescent clinic patients. *Arch Pediatr Adolesc Med.* 2002;156(6):607–614
3. Knight JR. *Substance Use, Abuse, and Dependence.* Philadelphia, PA: WB Saunders; 1999
4. Prochaska JO, DiClemente CC. Stages of change in the modification of problem behaviors. *Prog Behav Modif.* 1992;28:183–218

5. Miller WR, Rollnick S. *Motivational Interviewing: Preparing People for Change.* 2nd ed. New York, NY: Guilford Press; 2002
6. Kokotailo PK, Gold MA. Motivational interviewing with adolescents. *Adolesc Med.* 2008;19(1): 54–68
7. Hingson R, Heeren T, Winter M. Age at drinking onset and alcohol dependence: age at onset, duration, and severity. *Arch Pediatr Adolesc Med.* 2006;160(7):739–746
8. American Psychiatric Association. *Diagnostic and Statistical Manual of Mental Disorders.* 4th ed. Washington DC: American Psychiatric Association; 1994

Adherence in Adolescents: A Review of the Literature

Marvin E. Belzer, MD*, Johanna Olson, MD

Division of Adolescent Medicine, Childrens Hospital Los Angeles, 4650 Sunset Boulevard, MS #2, Los Angeles, CA 90027, USA

Physicians are charged with the task of improving the health and well-being of their patients, and those physicians who treat adolescents interact with their teenaged patients in many different ways to achieve this goal. Typical interactions include promoting healthy behaviors (ie, health education on appropriate diet and exercise), counseling on reducing risky sexual or drug-use behaviors, prescribing interventions (ie, medications, special diets, physical therapy), referring for specialty care (including mental health treatment), and recommending future follow-up. Research has demonstrated that clinical outcomes are closely linked to patient adherence[1] and that adolescents commonly have difficulty adhering to physician recommendations.[2-4] Although the adolescent-specific cost of nonadherence in mortality, morbidity, and financial burden is unknown, it is estimated that half of all medication-related hospitalizations in the United States (all ages) are attributable to nonadherence and cost $100 billion a year.[5]

In this article we review adolescent adherence, including how to measure adherence, factors associated with adherence and nonadherence, interventions to improve adherence, and research findings on adherence in those with selected chronic health conditions such as HIV infection, organ transplant, asthma, contraception, and diabetes mellitus. It should be noted that the literature for adolescent adherence in patients with organ transplants and diabetes is extensive, spanning several decades, and forms the basis of this article. In the past decade, literature on adult (and to a lesser extent, adolescent) HIV medication adherence has led to a better understanding of how to conduct useful research.

DEFINITION OF ADHERENCE

In the medical literature, the terms "adherence" and "compliance" are used interchangeably. The use of "compliance" has fallen from favor because of the perception

---

*Corresponding author.
E-mail address: mbelzer@chla.usc.edu (M. E. Belzer).

that compliance implies a paternalistic health care system in which the physician prescribes the treatment, and the patients and family must follow this advice or be seen in a negative context described as noncompliant. For the remainder of this article, the term "adherence" will be used, which is defined as the extent to which a patient's behavior (taking medication, following diets, or executing lifestyle changes) coincides with medical or health advice.[6] Meichenbaum and Turk[7] added a requirement that the definition include "active, voluntary, collaborative involvement of patient (and family) in a mutually acceptable course of behavior to produce a desired preventative or therapeutic result." This definition implies a reasoned agreement in treatment among the patient, family, and physician.

The percentage of prescribed doses taken by the patient defines the level of medication adherence and is generally disease- or condition-dependent, on the basis of the threshold needed for therapeutic effect. In most cases, taking 80% of prescribed doses is considered adherent for conditions such as asthma or hypertension. Medication adherence to insulin for diabetes and antiretroviral agents for HIV infection requires higher rates of use for the benefits of the medication to be realized. Because of the rapid rate of mutation of the HIV virus, patients infected with HIV are generally required to take 95% of antiretroviral doses to be considered adherent. Determining acceptable levels of adherence to diets, or risk-reduction behaviors, is even more complex and specific to the individual intervention. Adherence levels are usually defined as number of doses taken divided the by number of doses prescribed over a set period of time. However, it can also be defined in other ways, including taking enough medication to get the desired therapeutic effect. This variable is confounded by the fact that there are many factors that influence therapeutic effect, including pharmacokinetics, absorption, and disease-related factors; for example, 1 asthmatic patient might require lower doses of inhaled corticosteroid for adequate control than would another patient.

Nonadherence to medications can take many forms:

1. prescription is never filled;
2. underdose;
3. overdose (occurs commonly with analgesia but can occur with any medication);
4. mistiming of doses; and
5. nonadherence to food requirements (many medications require the patient to take medicine on an empty or full stomach or even with specific meals, such as ones with low or high fat to ensure sufficient absorption).

Some studies have used complex variables for adherence, which include combinations of the factors described above. In addition, nonadherence is sometimes categorized as intentional or unintentional.

SCOPE OF THE PROBLEM

The average level of adherence varies significantly. Dunbar's[8] review of pediatric and adolescent adherence in 1983 discovered an adherence range of 10% to 80%, with 50% being the average. In the last 2 decades, adherence research in adolescents (and children) has shown little improvement in patients with a variety of chronic illnesses, including asthma,[9] HIV infection,[10,11] diabetes,[4] and organ transplantation.[2] Treatment of acute conditions[12] has fared no better than that of chronic conditions. Adherence to medications is not the only problem. Adherence to appointments for things such as treatment of acne is also difficult.[13] Although studies directly comparing adolescents with children or adults have been few, reviews have generally reported that adolescents tend to adhere less than older or younger age groups.[14]

MEASURES OF ADHERENCE

There are numerous ways to measure adherence. Both in clinical practice and research, these measures are divided into direct and indirect methods (Table 1). Direct methods include directly observed therapy (DOT), measurement of drug or drug metabolite levels in the blood or other body fluid, and measurement of a biological marker. These direct methods can be expensive and burdensome, and they have the potential to be manipulated by patients (eg, selectively taking medications right before blood samples are collected). Indirect methods of measuring adherence include the use of pill counts, self-reporting (including questionnaires), electronic medication monitors, measuring physiologic markers (eg, measuring heart rate of patients on β blockers), and assessing clinical response. Indirect measures are generally less expensive and burdensome but are subject to numerous biases. It is critically important to understand the various adherence measures when trying to assess adherence. Although there is little adherence literature specific to adolescents,[15] there are significant data regarding adults.[5] It should also be noted that much of the recent literature on adherence measures has come from adult HIV research.[16-20]

Direct Measures

Pill Counts

Patients are asked to bring in their medications, and providers count out the number of doses taken and divide by the expected number of doses to be taken since the last visit. This method is time intensive and subject to the possibility of patients dumping pills before appointments. The use of unannounced pill counts during home visits has been shown to be a much more reliable counting method but is impractical for clinical use.[21,22] Unannounced pill counts conducted by telephone may be a more logistically feasible method,[23] especially as a clinical tool when working with nonadherent populations.

Table 1
Methods of measuring adherence

Test	Advantages	Disadvantages
Direct methods		
Directly observed therapy	Most accurate	Patients can hide pills in the mouth and then discard them; impractical for routine use
Measurement of the level of medicine or metabolite in blood	Objective	Variations in metabolism and "white-coat adherence" can give a false impression of adherence; expensive
Measurement of the biologic marker in blood	Objective; in clinical trials, can also be used to measure placebo	Requires expensive quantitative assays and collection of bodily fluids
Indirect methods		
Patient questionnaires, patient self-reports	Simple; inexpensive; the most useful method in the clinical setting	Susceptible to error with increases in time between visits; results are easily distorted by the patient
Pill counts	Objective; quantifiable, and easy to perform	Data easily altered by the patient (eg, pill dumping)
Rates of prescription refills	Objective; easy to obtain data	A prescription refill is not equivalent to ingestion of medication; requires a closed pharmacy system
Assessment of the patient's clinical response	Simple; generally easy to perform	Factors other than medication adherence can affect clinical response
Electronic medication monitors	Precise; results are easily quantified; tracks patterns of taking medication	Expensive; requires return visits and downloading data from medication vials
Measurement of physiologic markers (eg, heart rate in patients taking beta-blockers)	Often easy to perform	Marker may be absent for other reasons (eg, increased metabolism, poor absorption, lack of response)
Patient diaries	Help to correct for poor recall	Easily altered by the patient
When the patient is a child, questionnaire for caregiver or teacher	Simple; objective	Susceptible to distortion

Reproduced with permission from: Osterberg L, Blaschke T. Adherence to medication. N Engl J Med. 2005;353(5):489.

Pharmacy Refills

This method involves contacting pharmacies to determine if patients regularly refill their medications. It is easy to perform but only works when the patient uses only 1 pharmacy and orders are not automatically shipped on a regular basis. This method assumes that prescriptions filled are taken, and that patients who are not refilling prescriptions are not filling them at other pharmacies and, hence, are considered nonadherent. Although this method is far from perfect, it avoids the social-desirability and response bias in most other methods.

Drug and Metabolite Levels

Therapeutic drug monitoring is feasible in most clinical and research settings for which assays have been developed. Some drug assays are very expensive. In addition, there are many factors that can affect drug levels, including absorption, food effects, and drug-drug interactions. It is also common for patients to take their medications just before appointments in an attempt to falsely indicate adherence. Tests that validate long-term adherence include the measurement of hemoglobin A1C levels and the use of glucose-monitoring devices that store glucose-level data.

Indirect Measures

Electronic Drug Monitoring

This method is generally considered the gold standard by adherence researchers because of its ability to validate results for a variety of adult diseases.[16,24,25] The most studied device is the medication event monitoring system cap. The device, which looks like a bottle cap, has a microprocessor that monitors and stores the time and date each time the bottle is opened. One benefit of this method is that it includes the time that medication is taken. Potential problems include curiosity opening on the part of a patient (leads to overestimating adherence) and the pocketing of extra doses for later use (leads to underestimation of adherence). In addition, patients are clearly aware that their adherence is being monitored and can open the cap without taking medication. Medication event monitoring system devices are usually large, and youth are frequently unwilling to take them along when they leave their home, thus making them only suitable for use when all medications are used exclusively at home. Some newer devices have alarms built in[26] and act as both an adherence intervention and measuring device.

Self-report

This is the most common measure of adherence used in both clinical and research settings. There is less burden on medical staff, and it is inexpensive. Patients can also be asked to identify the reasons why they missed doses of medication so that patient-specific interventions can be developed within a clinical setting. Self-reporting has been reviewed and is considered quite valid in adult HIV studies.[17,18,27] The vast majority of studies have demonstrated good correlation between self-reporting and several direct measures including electronic drug monitoring and HIV RNA reductions (biological marker of effective HIV treatment). In adolescents with HIV, self-report data correlated well with HIV RNA reductions (biological marker) in 1 cohort study.[10] Disadvantages of self-reporting include the lack of standardized questions, social-response and recall bias, and a general finding that patients overestimate adherence.[16] One unresolved methodologic issue in self-reporting adherence involves choosing an optimal time frame for recall periods. Recall periods can be 1, 3, 7, or 30 days or may be yesterday or last weekend. Although shorter periods may reduce recall bias, longer periods may have better associations with disease outcomes. There are several techniques for reducing the social-response bias that may lead studies to overestimate adherence. Most questionnaires now state up front that it is difficult to have 100% adherence, and that most people miss some doses. Some researchers find that patients may give more accurate information if the data are collected by using a computer-assisted self-interview or paper and pencil as opposed to direct staff interview. Computer-assisted self-interviews can also use an audio component that reduces the issue of literacy (or lack of it) being a factor. Another popular tool in collecting self-report data is to replace Likert scales (eg, scores of 1–7) with visual analog scales.[28,29]

Summary of Adherence Measurements

Although all research measures have their benefits and faults, there is no current gold standard for measuring adherence.[19] Simoni et al[17] have suggested (within the HIV field) that "both researchers and clinicians may proceed with the use of self-report measures. Intervention trials may have better validation if less subjective measures such as electronic data monitoring or pill counts are used." Research specific to adherence may be best accomplished if at least 2 measures of adherence are used. Composite adherence measures that use several different standards may be a good compromise.[16] Clinicians must always be aware that self-report results may be false and that tools such as pill counts or pharmacy-refill data can be misleading. Nothing can replace good clinical acumen that includes a trusting doctor-patient relationship, measures of adherence that may include self-reporting, pill counts, pharmacy refills, or therapeutic drug levels, and the synthesis of these results in conjunction with expected clinical outcomes.

Barriers to Adherence for Adolescents

The World Health Organization has placed factors that affect adherence into 5 interrelated categories.[1]

Demographic and Socioeconomic Factors

In general, most studies have not found race, ethnicity, gender, or poverty to have independent links to nonadherence in adolescents. Although the age of an adolescent (early adolescence: [12–14 years old] versus late adolescence: [18–21 years old]) has yet to be consistently linked to nonadherence, adolescents as a whole have been found to be less adherent than children or adults in some studies. Socioeconomic factors related to family dynamics have been barriers to adherence. Lack of parental supervision or support has been linked to nonadherence in patients after receiving a renal transplant[30] and in diabetic adolescents.[31] Lack of active parental involvement in treatment, atmosphere of family conflict, and even single-parent households have been linked to nonadherence.[2]

Treatment-Related Factors

A number of factors related to the complexity of the treatment regimen have been related to adherence. These factors include the number of medications prescribed, the total number of pills, pill size, and pill taste. Some teenagers (especially young ones) have yet to learn to swallow pills, and this factor makes large pill size or bad pill taste particularly burdensome. Taking medications once a day is somewhat better than twice a day, but adherence is markedly better than ≥3 times per day.[32] Food requirements make adherence more complicated as well. Longer length of treatment has been linked to nonadherence.[9,33] Adverse effects have consistently been linked to nonadherence. From short-term adverse effects such as gastrointestinal upset to longer-term and more severe adverse effects such as body disfigurement from long-term use of corticosteroid or HIV medications are important detriments to taking medications. Contraception adherence is closely linked to both adverse effects (abnormal bleeding and weight gain) and the length of time on hormones.[33] Adolescents with other barriers such as poor physician-patient relationship or mental illness may be extremely unwilling to deal with even mild transient adverse effects, which makes comprehensive education before initiating treatment critical.

Condition-Related Factors

Little is known about how the severity, chronicity, or persistence of a particular illness impacts adherence. Although one might intuitively think that more severely ill/symptomatic youth would be more adherent, at least 1 study in HIV-infected adolescents linked advanced disease status to nonadherence.[11] Clearly, nonadherence can be linked to deteriorating health in conditions such as HIV, organ transplant, malignancy, and diabetes so that one must be careful in interpreting this linkage. It is not hard to imagine how frustration and self-efficacy could be altered in more severely ill youth in whom the use of medications may not bring significant or immediate relief and might, thus, be linked to nonadherence. Diseases that have no symptoms, such as hypertension, hypercholesterolemia, or even early HIV, may lead youth (with little long-term focus) to judge treatment as unnecessary. Adolescents with chronic diseases will often experiment with a stretch of nonadherence, even after years of impeccable adherence to judge the balance between the disease process and the burden of the treatment.[34] Adolescents who are asymptomatic for long periods of time are less motivated to take their medications, and they do not maintain their lifestyle changes, because the immediate benefits of medication are not clearly obvious.

Health Care Setting and Health Care Provider Factors

Factors as simple as access to continuous insurance are important, because dropped coverage leads to nonadherence to appointments and medications. Economically disadvantaged families may be especially susceptible to this barrier, because their complex lives, limited education, and poor access to transportation may prevent them from regular access to public benefits. In today's complex insurance environment, frequent changes to insurance plans can block access to past providers or previously used medications, which poses a barrier to adherence. Timely authorization and delivery of medications to patients are frequently interrupted during changes in medical insurance or the provider.

One of the single-most important factors to patient adherence is the patient-provider relationship. In a qualitative review of pediatric adherence, Wolf et al[35] identified lack of time with provider (44%), insufficient information (40%), feeling of dependence (40%), no communication about adherence (34%), and loss of trust in doctors (33%) as the most common factors that affect adherence. Another study found that clinic visits that interfere with school or social functions might isolate patients from their peers and lead to nonadherence.[36] Studies have revealed that 50% of patients leave the office unsure of what they have been told.[24,34] Physicians who fail to provide adequate time, frequent visits, good listening skills, and appropriate education are creating an atmosphere that may lead to a lack of trust or respect for the clinician. Although demonstrating compassion and empathy may be difficult in a health care system that rewards short and rushed visits, it nonetheless may reinforce powerful negative messages to patients and their families that can be directly linked to poor health outcomes.

Patient-Related Factors

Particularly for adolescents, barriers to medication adherence are intricately enmeshed with the developmental challenges that young people face during this time of transition. The development of a child to an adolescent and then into an adult is a complex process that involves rapid changes in the development of both the body and the brain. This process is even more complicated in children with chronic illness in whom development may be impaired or delayed. Cognitive delay, even when mild, may require lifelong support in regards to medication adherence. Several normal adolescent development processes may seriously interfere with adherence. The normal process of separation and individuation leads adolescents to exert control over their lives. One opportunity to exert this independence from parents is to control medication adherence. Youth with parental conflict may choose to be intentionally nonadherent. Some parents (with or without abnormal conflict) may prematurely pass the responsibility of taking medications to their children before they are really ready. Other important developmental factors are feelings of invulnerability and lack of interest in the future. Some youth, even with potentially life-threatening illnesses, will see taking medication as a low priority as compared with the need for fitting in with their peers. The most common reasons cited by youth for missing doses of medication include forgetting, leaving home without medication, and changing daily routine.[37,38] Youth concerned about fitting in with their peers render adverse effects such as weight gain or change in skin appearance intolerable.[39] Some youth will refuse to take medications at school or miss school for fear that peers will know they are ill.

Many adolescents who develop chronic health conditions have little past experience managing health issues. Of more concern are those who enter the health care system with misconceptions based on childhood experiences (ie, painful immunizations), their parents' prejudices, or lack of trust. In 1 adult HIV study, black men were found to be more negative in terms of their belief in their physician's expertise and in their ability to adhere.[40] Events such as the Tuskegee experiments with syphilis[41], more general experiences of cultural insensitivity, or frank prejudice from past health care providers mold initial relationships and require significant attention to maximize adherence. Youths' lack of knowledge may lead to a lack of understanding of how medications work and how missing medications relates to the severity of illness or its progression. Many interventions to improve adherence (discussed later) focus on this lack of knowledge and the need to improve a patient's sense of personal control over their illness. The concept that improved self-efficacy ("I have the ability to regularly take medication") and outcome expectancy ("taking medication will improve my health") improve adherence are a focus of current adolescent research.

Psychosocial factors are critical in their impact on adherence. Mental illness, especially depression, has been linked to adolescent nonadherence with HIV treatment[10] and diabetes.[42] Patient anger has been linked to nonadherence in patients after renal transplants[43] and is likely to be an important factor in many chronic debilitating illnesses. Posttraumatic stress disorder with or without childhood abuse is thought to impact adherence[44] and is an active area for research. Substance misuse and abuse is another factor that leads to nonadherence in adolescents[11] and is likely a major factor for some patients.

ADHERENCE INTERVENTIONS

Unfortunately, there have been very few well-designed and successful randomized clinical trials that examined how best to intervene with nonadherent youth. Strategies to improve adherence are generally divided into regimen-simplification/adverse-effect management, improving the patient-provider relationship, educational strategies, behavioral strategies, counseling techniques, referrals for mental health and substance abuse treatment, and DOT. Some of these interventions have been clearly tested, whereas others address issues of patient nonadherence and can be seen as promising practices. Not all of these interventions have been derived from studies with adolescents; instead, they were derived from study results with adults.

Regimen Simplification/Adverse Effects

Patients almost always have improved adherence with simpler and better-tolerated medications/interventions. Medications should be given no more than once or twice daily. Medication regimens must be compatible with the youth's schedule, acknowledging that medication food requirements must fit into what may be an erratic dietary schedule. Timing of medication must fit into school, work, and social activities, which include evening and weekend events. Many youth do not wish their peers to know about their medical conditions, which may lead to the avoidance of taking medication during school or other social activities. Some teenagers (especially younger teenagers) are frustrated by having to take large pills, large numbers of pills, or medications that do not taste good. Practitioners need to explore these factors with their patients and families and design a simple regimen that fits the needs of the patient. A trial run for 2 to 3 weeks that uses practice medications may help teenagers handle some of the barriers that come up in day-to-day life and assist them in choosing a practical regimen. At times, it may be necessary to choose a suboptimal treatment strategy if the likelihood for a better outcome on the basis of improved adherence is probable. For example, a parent might avoid giving children medicine at bedtime if they frequently miss doses at night because they inadvertently fall asleep or have a tendency to stay out late with friends and may not even come home some nights. Another example may involve avoiding inhalers and only using pills for some asthmatic patients who are averse to inhaler use. Many adolescents will not tolerate adverse effects, especially if those are worse than their disease-related symptoms in the short run. The development of diarrhea during school or work is often intolerable. Adverse effects that affect a patient's appearance are frequently troublesome.[40] Patients who have received a transplant may stop using corticosteroids because of the development of cushingoid features. Patients with HIV can develop facial and extremity fat loss, which is both disfiguring and likely to lead to inadvertent disclosure of their illness. Care must be taken to educate youth and their families about potential adverse effects, prearrange plans for how these adverse effects will be managed, and display a willingness to quickly change regimens if the adverse effects are intolerable to the patient.

Patient-Provider Relationship

One key to improving patient adherence involves the development of a trusting and supportive relationship between patients and their providers. This may start with providers speaking directly to youth as opposed to speaking exclusively to their parents. They may need to ask the parents to leave for part of the visit to explore confidential issues. Frequent visits can assist in relationship building and facilitate the practitioner's understanding of how the patient's illness and medication use fit into or adversely affect their patient's lives. Friendly office staff and shorter waiting times can also improve the quality of the patient-provider relationship.

Educational Strategies

Although patient and family education concerning illness is considered a critical factor in promoting adherence,[40,45] research results for adults, including meta-analyses, have concluded that educational strategies alone are not sufficient.[46,47] Adolescents need to know the purpose of and schedules for their treatment plans. They need to understand and buy into the fact that their medications may need to be taken with certain food requirements (ie, that some medication may not be absorbed unless taken on a full or empty stomach or that they may cause increased adverse effects if taken on an empty stomach). Adolescents need to understand the short-term and long-term consequences of taking or missing their prescribed treatments (ie, diabetic patients need to understand that missing meals may lead to hypoglycemia, iron-deficient girls may be fatigued or could perform worse in school if they avoid treatment, youth with HIV may develop severe resistance to antiretroviral medications if adherence is inconsistent, or a patient who received a renal transplant may face organ rejection and need dialysis because of nonadherence). Verbal education can be augmented with written materials or educational videos. It is critical to use educational strategies that incorporate a patient's developmental and cognitive abilities. Less cognitively developed adolescents who are concrete thinkers need specific and clear directions about the short-term aspects of their treatment plans. Education needs to be repeated at each visit, plans need to be adjusted according to life changes and reiterated at each visit, and patients should be encouraged to ask questions.

Behavioral Strategies

There are many behavioral strategies that can be used to assist patients with adherence.[2] The use of practice medications can help an adolescent get used to the routine of taking medication before they start taking real medication. In most cases, it is best to avoid the use of candy placebos, because this provides a reward that will not be replicated with the actual medication. Youth can use calendars, diaries, or pocket computers to record and, thus, reinforce use of their treatment. Reminders for taking medications can come from alarms, pagers, cellular phones, or even the parent. Cues are very helpful as reminders, and they include taking medications at meals and putting the medication next to a toothbrush or razor. The use of pill boxes can help remind those youth who forget if they have already taken their medication as they work through their busy schedules. The use of rewards is a common behavioral method for helping youth get used to the routine of taking their medications. Rewards can include gifts, points, praise, privileges, or even cash. In general, rewards cannot be used in perpetuity; the goal should eventually be to link adherence to positive self-esteem.

Counseling Techniques

It is appealing to use counseling to address some of the common barriers to adherence, which include depression, substance abuse, poor social support, low self-efficacy or self-esteem, or other individual mental health problems that deter adherence. The literature on diabetic patients contains the largest number of randomized clinical trials that used both individual and group counseling for adolescents; however, meta-analysis results have only shown modest improvements in metabolic control.[48] Adult HIV literature reviews have indicated some benefits from the use of cognitive behavioral therapy (CBT) or individualized counseling interventions.[49,50] CBT targets faulty belief systems, thoughts, and behaviors that interfere with goals and maintain problem behaviors. Teaching coping skills and relapse prevention are also tenets of CBT.[51] Motivational interviewing is a client-centered, goal-directed counseling style originally developed to treat substance abuse and was later adapted to facilitate a broader range of social and behavioral changes.[52] Motivational interviewing includes 5 counseling techniques aimed at helping clients resolve ambivalence about a health behavior: (1) expressing empathy; (2) developing discrepancy; (3) avoiding argument; (4) rolling with resistance (avoid being overly confrontational if patient expresses resistance to change); and (5) supporting self-efficacy.[53] Motivational interviewing is based on the premise that a patient's readiness for change is not fixed but fluctuates and can be altered through this type of intervention. A pilot study of motivational interviewing to improve adult adherence to HIV medications has demonstrated feasibility,[54] and a randomized, clinical trial in adolescents is currently in process.

Mental Health and Substance Abuse Treatment Referral

Many study results have demonstrated that mental health disorders (especially depression) and substance abuse reduce adherence. Although the counseling interventions mentioned above may assist these patients, more focused treatment by psychiatrists, psychologists, therapists, and substance abuse programs (including detoxification, residential treatment, individual, and 12-step programs) are required. Once mental health conditions are stabilized, then adherence may benefit from the other techniques described above. Children with oppositional defiant, conduct disorders, or just a chaotic nonsupportive home environment may require placement in a group home, foster care, or treatment facility to adequately address life-threatening nonadherence (ie, organ transplant rejection, advanced AIDS-related illnesses, cancer treatment, or recurrent admission for diabetic ketoacidosis).

Directly Observed Therapy

DOT was originally designed for nonadherent patients who required treatment for tuberculosis. It involves a provider directly observing a patient taking his or her medications. DOT is quite intensive and expensive and requires an outreach worker to visit the patient on a daily basis. DOT has been quite successful both nationally and internationally in improving treatment outcomes and reducing the development of multiresistant strains of tuberculosis. Because of similar concerns with the development of resistance to HIV medications, several studies have explored the use of DOT. These tend to be successful when linked to an institutionalized living system (eg, jail) or a methadone-maintenance program. A pilot study for youth with HIV is currently in progress, but the impracticality of this intervention may preclude its use in all but the most extreme situations. One common form of DOT involves the direct participation of parents and guardians. Golden et al[55] found that direct parental involvement in giving or observing insulin injections reduced admission rates for ketoacidosis. This level of support can be critical for some patients, but for others, issues of previous poor parenting, the developmental tasks of separation and individuation, and search for autonomy may lead to severe parent-youth discord over adherence. In these cases, the use of individual and family counseling may be needed. In extreme cases, placement out of the home may be critical for preventing severe morbidity or mortality. In general, parental participation with youth adherence is important, and supervision should not be abruptly terminated but, instead, gradually reduced as the youth demonstrates competence. In addition, because adherence typically waxes and wanes over time, even adherent youth need some level of support and supervision to maintain adherence.

ADOLESCENT ADHERENCE IN SPECIFIC DISEASES

Adolescents with chronic conditions including asthma, transplants, diabetes, and HIV stand to suffer serious consequences as a result of nonadherence to both lifestyle changes and medication regimens. These consequences include advancement of the disease process, decline in physical functioning, increased time in the hospital, and increased morbidity and mortality rates.[34]

HIV

Adherence is a particularly unique and difficult challenge for youth infected with HIV because of the fact that ≥95% adherence to highly active antiretroviral therapy is required to achieve adequate viral suppression and avoid development of resistance.[24] In addition, many young people with HIV (infected both perinatally and behaviorally) often face additional challenges with respect to family structure and support, drug use, poverty, and stigmatization of their illness. Youth infected with HIV have been recognized to have difficulties with keeping appointments[56] and taking medications.[10,57] The most detailed information on medication adherence comes from the prospective, longitudinal, observational, multisite Reaching for Excellence in Adolescent Care and Health study.[58] In this longitudinal study, 325 behaviorally infected youth with HIV were recruited before the age of 19 and followed every 3 months. Nearly 75% of the youth were female, and 76% of the female youth and 60% of the male youth identified as black. Murphy and colleagues[10,11,36] have published 3 articles that described adherence in this cohort. They found that only 41% reported full adherence by the self-report method in the previous month. Self-reported adherence was associated with reductions in HIV RNA by polymerase chain reaction (viral load). Nonadherence was associated with depression, and a trend toward decreased adherence was also associated with increased numbers of medications prescribed. Barriers to adherence were analyzed by factor analysis, and medication-related adverse effects (both physical and psychological) and complications in day-to-day routines accounted for the largest proportion of variance. The most common reasons cited for missing medication doses included reports that the youth "simply forgot" (46%), "did not have medication with me" (42%), and changed "daily routines" (33%). Some of the other issues cited by the subjects included "did not want others to notice medications, did not like taste, too many pills, reminds me I have HIV or felt depressed or overwhelmed." Longitudinal adherence was analyzed in 65 initially adherent subjects whose progress was followed for ~1 year. Median time to nonadherence was 12 months. Subjects with more advanced HIV illness were less adherent. Less alcohol use and being in school were associated with improved adherence on weekends and in the preceding month. Failure to maintain adherence was associated with younger age and depression. Adherence of this cohort is clearly troublesome, and interventions to improve adherence are currently in study or in development, but there has been no research that has defined the interventions that would be most useful. Another study that documented the problems with adolescent adherence came from the Pediatric AIDS Clinical Trails Group study of virological and immunologic outcomes of adolescents on highly active antiretroviral therapy.[59] Complete adherence over the first 24 weeks of this 3-year study was only 27%. The 3-year results have been submitted for publication, and it is troublesome that only 37% of the cohort remained on study treatment for the full 3 years, and only 24% maintained undetectable HIV RNA levels for the duration of the study (the optimal treatment outcome). Maintenance of undetectable viral load was associated with medication adherence. With the goal of lifelong viral suppression of HIV and the understanding that suboptimal adherence and viral suppression leads to permanent viral resistance, it is clear that research for appropriate interventions will be a priority for researchers of adolescent HIV.

Organ Transplant

The risk of morbidity and mortality is high among adolescents who receive organ transplants. Nonadherence with immunosuppressive medications is associated with an increased risk of late-acute graft rejection and was reviewed by Dobbels et al in 2005.[2] This review noted that adolescents have poorer long-term outcomes than children or adults. Nonadherence was common regardless of which measures were used (41.8% for pill counts, 36.5% for self-report, 24.8% for cyclosporine levels, and 21% for electronic drug monitoring). Risk factors for nonadherence parallel those of other medical conditions. Both intentional and unintentional nonadherence occurs, and intentional nonuse is often associated with the disfiguring adverse effects of immunosuppressive medications. One study of adolescents and young adults revealed that immaturity was a strong predictor of nonadherence.[60] There has been a complete lack of randomized, clinical trials that have evaluated interventions to improve on adherence in adolescent transplant recipients. The foundation of clinical intervention is based on educational strategies that promote a better understanding of disease and treatment, behavioral strategies that include diaries, pill boxes, alarms, rewards for correct dosing, the use of cues to remind patients to take medications, and, finally, to improve social support (including active involvement of parents and guardians).

Asthma

Asthma is one of the most common illnesses in adolescence, and nonadherence to treatment has been documented to lead to increased morbidity rates, especially in terms of increased hospitalizations. Nonadherence to medications is common,[9,37,61] and it generally worsens over time. Open communication with teenagers is critical in the education process, and it also allows for ownership of their health status. Education must include the avoidance of triggers such as dust, pollen, viral infections, and, most importantly, exposure to tobacco smoke (either active or passive.) Despite a common desire for adolescents to establish and maintain autonomy around medication regimens, parental involvement is usually beneficial. It is also common for adolescents to be concerned about taking medications at school (embarrassment) so that the use of once- or twice-daily medications, which can be taken exclusively at home, is optimal. Intervening by use of personalized treatment plans designed to include chronic treatment and treatment of exacerbations is favored.

Contraception

Poor adherence to hormonal contraception (reviewed by Clark[33]) must be divided into missing doses of prescribed medication and premature discontinuation (which technically is not nonadherent because women often make a conscious decision to terminate use). After 3 months of use, only 44% to 45% of adolescents are adherent to oral contraceptive pills (OCPs), and this number drops to 33% at the end of 1 year. This decrease leads to high failure rates (unintended pregnancies) of 25% to 50%. Research has found that adverse effects and fear of adverse effects are the most common reasons for terminating the use of OCPs. Approximately half of discontinuations occur because of breakthrough bleeding, although nausea, headaches, amenorrhea, and weight gain are other common reasons. There is some concern that preferred use of low-dose OCPs leads to more breakthrough bleeding than previous formulations and could lead to more disuse. Discontinuation of Depo Provera is also common (47%–78% at the end of 1 year) and usually linked to adverse effects as well. To evaluate how adherence to hormonal contraception is related to health concerns, Clark[33] reviewed relevant studies from 1980 to 2000 and found that misconceptions about contraceptives and adverse effects were the most pressing problems. Although the quality of existing research does not provide strong guidance as to the best interventions,[62] most experts recommend better education on the use, expected adverse effects, and their management to improve adherence and prevent premature discontinuation. Education of parents may also be of value, given the findings that parental acceptance of adolescent sexuality[63] or teenagers' relationship with their mother's predicted use of birth control.[64]

Diabetes Mellitus

Adolescents with diabetes are one of the most challenging populations when it comes to adherence. Youth with diabetes have intense requirements for insulin therapy, glucose monitoring, dietary and exercise management, and appointment keeping. Diabetes is fairly unique among chronic diseases in youth in that the direct outcome measures of adherence, including hemoglobin A1C and computerized glucose monitoring devices with memory, are standard. The literature for adherence to diabetic care is quite robust and was last reviewed (for type 1 diabetes) by Hoffman[4] in 2002. The outcomes of poor adherence include short-term complications of increased hospitalizations for diabetic ketoacidosis and long-term complications such as retinal and renal disease. Major psychiatric disorders that develop after the onset of diabetes are predictors of future nonadherence.[41] Lack of parental involvement has also been reported to cause poor adherence.[31] Reductions in insulin use may also occur in those youth who desire weight loss. Interventions to improve adherence to diabetes treatment have had mixed results. A meta-analysis of 18 studies showed that behavioral interventions lead to modest improvements in glycosylated hemoglobin (0.3%–0.6%).[47] Parental or family-member supervision that incorporates directly observed insulin therapy, psychotherapy, and even threatened or actual placement of youth outside the home have been found to end strings of admissions for diabetic ketoacidosis caused by poor adherence.[54,65] More recent studies have indicated that self-efficacy may be linked to adherence[66] and that intensive, home-based psychotherapy (multisystemic therapy) improves adherence in type 1 diabetic patients.[67] The need for similar research for the expanding population of type 2 diabetic adolescents is needed, because adherence has clearly been linked with metabolic control.[68]

Table 2
Recommendations for Clinicians

Regimen simplification
  Minimize dosing frequency, pill number and size
  Fit regimen into youth's schedule
  Utilize forgiving regimen
Adherence assessment
  Assess adherence clinically at all visits
  Utilize questionnaire
  Address barriers if nonadherent
Enhance communication
  Schedule frequent appointments
  Allow adequate time for patient and family education
  Meet individually with teen if confidentiality needed
Cues
  Identify cues (like meals, shaving, brushing teeth) to taking medications
Psychosocial problems
  Regularly assess for social/family support, mental illness, substance abuse and refer as needed

CONCLUSIONS

Adolescent adherence is an extremely complex challenge, and nonadherence is a clear risk factor for poor health outcomes. Although there has been extensive research exploring how to measure adherence and which factors influence adherence, there has been relatively little research to demonstrate useful interventions for the practicing clinician. It is likely that future research will demonstrate the need for multiple interventions for each patient. On the basis of current clinical consensus, Table 2 delineates suggestions for improving adherence in adolescents.

REFERENCES

1. Sabate E. Adherence to long-term therapies: evidence for action. Available at: www.who.int/chp/knowledge/publications/adherence_report/en/index.html. Accessed March 14, 2008
2. Dobbels F, Van Damme-Lombaert R, Vanhaecke J, De Geest S. Growing pains: nonadherence with the immunosuppressive regimen in adolescent transplant recipients. *Pediatr Transplant*. 2005;9(3):381–390
3. Nevins TE. Why do they do that? The compliance conundrum. *Pediatr Nephrol*. 2005;20(7): 845–848
4. Hoffman RP. Adolescent adherence in type 1 diabetes. *Compr Ther*. 2002;28(2):128–133
5. Osterberg L, Blaschke T. Adherence to medication. *N Engl J Med*. 2005;353(5):487–497
6. Haynes RB, Taylor DW, Sackett DL, eds. *Compliance in Health Care* . Baltimore, MD: Johns Hopkins University Press; 1979:1–70
7. Meichenbaum D, Turk DC. Treatment adherence: terminology, incidence and conceptualization. In: Meichenbaum D, Turk DC, eds. *Facilitating Treatment Adherence* . New York, NY: Plenum Press; 1987:19–39
8. Dunbar J. Compliance in pediatrics populations: a review. In: McGraph PJ, Fireston P, eds. *Pediatric and Adolescent Behavioral Medicine: Issues in Treatment* . New York, NY: Springer; 1983

9. Jónasson G, Carlsen K, Mowinckel P. Asthma drug adherence in a long-term clinical trial. *Arch Dis Child.* 2000;83(4):330–333
10. Murphy DA, Wilson CM, Durako SJ, Muenz LR, Belzer M; Adolescent Medicine HIV/AIDS Research Network. Antiretroviral medication adherence among the REACH HIV-infected adolescent cohort in the USA. *AIDS Care.* 2001;13(1):27–40
11. Murphy DA, Belzer M, Durako SJ, et al. Longitudinal antiretroviral adherence among adolescents infected with human immunodeficiency virus. *Arch Pediatr Adolesc Med.* 2005;159(8): 764–770
12. Cromer BA, Steinberg K, Gardner L, Thornton D, Shannon B. Psychosocial determinants of compliance in adolescents with iron deficiency. *Am J Dis Child.* 1989;143(1):55–58
13. McEvoy B, Nydegger R, Wiliams G. Factors related to patient compliance in the treatment of acne vulgaris. *Int J Dermatol.* 2003;42(4):274–280
14. Costello I, Wong IC, Nunn AJ. A literature review to identify interventions to improve the use of medicines in children. *Child Care Health Dev.* 2004;30(6):647–665
15. Wiener L, Riekert K, Ryder C, Wood LV. Assessing medication adherence in adolescents with HIV when electronic monitoring is not feasible. *AIDS Patient Care STDS.* 2004;18(9):527–538
16. Berg KM, Arnsten JH. Practical and conceptual challenges in measuring antiretroviral adherence. *J Acquir Immune Defic Syndr.* 2006;43(suppl 1):S79–S87
17. Simoni JM, Kurth AE, Pearson CR, Pantalone DW, Merrill JO, Frick PA. Self-report measures of antiretroviral therapy adherence: a review with recommendations for HIV research and clinical management. *AIDS Behav.* 2006;10(3):227–245
18. Pearson CR, Simoni JM, Hoff P, Kurth AE, Martin DP. Assessing antiretroviral adherence via electronic drug monitoring and self-report: an examination of key methodological issues. *AIDS Behav.* 2007;11(2):161–173
19. Chesney MA. The elusive gold standard: future perspectives for HIV adherence assessment and intervention. *J Acquir Immune Defic Syndr.* 2006;43(suppl 1):S149–S155
20. Garber MC, Nau DP, Erikson SR, Aikens JE, Lawrence JB. The concordance of self-report with other measures of medication adherence. *Med Care.* 2004;42(7):649–652
21. Bangsberg DR, Hecht FM, Charlebois ED, Chesney M, Moss A. Comparing objective measures of adherence to HIV antiretroviral therapy: electronic medication monitoring and unannounced pill counts. *AIDS Behav.* 2001;5(3):275–281
22. Moss AR, Hahn JA, Perry S, et al. Adherence to highly active antiretroviral therapy in the homeless population in San Francisco: a prospective study. *Clin Infect Dis.* 2004;39(8):1190–1198
23. Kalichman SC, Amaral CM, Stearns H, et al. Adherence to antiretroviral therapy assessed by unannounced pill counts conducted by telephone. *J Gen Intern Med.* 2007;22(7):1003–1006
24. Cramer JA. Microeletronic systems for monitoring and enhancing patient compliance with medication regimens. *Drugs.* 1995;49(3):321–327
25. Rosen MI, Rigsby MO, Salahi JT, Ryan CE, Cramer JA. Electronic monitoring and counseling to improve medication adherence. *Behav Res Ther.* 2004;42(4):409–422
26. Wu AW, Snyder CF, Huang A, et al. A randomized trial of the impact of a programmable medication reminder device on quality of life in patients with AIDS. *AIDS Patient Care STDS.* 2006;20(11):773–781
27. Nieuwkerk PT, Oort FJ. Self-reported adherence to antiretroviral therapy for HIV-1 infection and virologic treatment response: a meta-analysis. *J Acquir Immune Defic Syndr.* 2005;38(4):445–448
28. Giordano TP, Guzman D, Clark R, Charlebois ED, Bangsberg DR. Measuring adherence to antiretroviral therapy in a diverse population using a visual analogue scale. *HIV Clin Trials.* 2004;5(2):74–79
29. Walsh JC, Mandalia S, Gazzard BG. Responses to a 1 month self-report on adherence to antiretroviral therapy are consistent with electronic data and virological treatment outcome. *AIDS.* 2002;16(2):269–277
30. Foulkes LM, Boggs SR, Fennell RS, Skibinski K. Social support, family variables, and compliance in renal transplant children. *Pediatr Nephrol.* 1993;7(2):185–188

31. Wysocki T, Meinhold PA, Abrams KC, et al. Parental and professional estimates of self-care independence of children and adolescents with IDDM. *Diabetes Care.* 1992;15(1):43–52
32. Eldred LJ, Wu AW, Chaisson RE, Moore RD. Adherence to antiretroviral and pneumocystis prophylaxis in HIV disease. *J Acquir Immune Defic Syndr Hum Retrovirol.* 1998;18(2):117–125
33. Clark LR. Will the pill make me sterile? Addressing reproductive health concerns and strategies to improve adherence to hormonal contraceptive regimens in adolescent girls. *J Pediatr Adolesc Gynecol.* 2001;14(4):153–162
34. Smith BA, Schuman M. Problem of nonadherence in chronically ill adolescents: strategies for assesment and intervention. *Curr Opin Pediatr.* 2005;17(5):613–618
35. Wolff BA, Strecker K, Vester U, Latta K, Ehrich JH. Noncompliance following renal transplantation in children and adolescents. *Pediatr Nephrol.* 1998;12(9):703–708
36. Warady BA, Mudge C, Wiser B, Wiser M, Rader B. Transplant allograft loss in the adolescent patient. *Adv Ren Replace Ther.* 1996;3(2):154–165
37. Murphy DA, Sarr M, Durako SJ, et al. Barriers to HAART adherence among human immunodeficiency virus-infected adolescents. *Arch Pediatr Adolesc Med.* 2003;157(3):249–155
38. Buston KM, Wood SF. Noncompliance amongst adolescents with asthma: listening to what they tell us about self-management. *Fam Pract.* 2000;17(2):134–138
39. Korsch BM, Fine RN, Negrete VF. Noncompliance in children with renal transplants. *Pediatrics.* 1978;61(6):872–876
40. Siegel K, Karus S, Schrimshaw EW. Racial differences in attitudes toward protease inhibitors among older HIV-infected men. *AIDS Care.* 2000;12(4):423–434
41. White RM. Misinformation and misbeliefs in the Tuskegee Study of Untreated Syphilis fuel mistrust in the healthcare system. *J Natl Med Assoc.* 2005;97(11):1566–1573
42. Kovacs M, Goldston D, Obrosky S, Ivengar S. Prevalence and predictors of pervasive noncompliance with medical treatment among youth with insulin-dependent diabetes mellitus. *J Am Acad Child Adolesc Psychiatry.* 1992;31(6):1112–1119
43. Penkower L, Dew MA, Ellis D, Sereika SM, Kitutu JM, Shapiro R. Psychological distress and adherence to the medical regimen among adolescent renal transplant recipients. *Am J Transplant.* 2003;3(11):1418–1425
44. Shemesh E, Lurie S, Stuber ML, et al. A pilot study of posttraumatic stress and nonadherence in pediatric liver transplant recipients. *Pediatrics.* 2000;105(2). Available at: www.pediatrics.org/cgi/content/full/105/2/e29
45. Griffin KJ, Elkin TD. Nonadherence in pediatric transplantation: a review of the literature. *Pediatr Transplant.* 2001;5(4):246–249
46. Roter DL, Hall JA, Merisca R, Nordstrom B, Cretin D, Svarstad B. Effectiveness of interventions to improve patient compliance: a meta-analysis. *Med Care.* 1998;36(8):1138–1161
47. Haynes RB, Montague P, Oliver T, et al. Interventions for helping patients to follow prescriptions for medication [Cochrane review]. In: *The Cochrane Library* . Issue 4. Oxford, United Kingdom: Update Software; 2000
48. Hampson SE, Skinner TC, Hart J, et al. Behavioral interventions for adolescents with type 1 diabetes. *Diabetes Care.* 2000;23(9):1416–1422
49. Simoni JM, Pantalone DW, Frick PA, Turner BJ. Enhancing antiretroviral adherence: a review of published reports of randomized controlled trials and on-going NIH-funded research. In: Trafton JA, Gordon WP, eds. *Best Practices in the Behavioral Management of Chronic Disease 2006.* Vol 2. Los Altos, CA: Institute for Disease Management; 2007
50. Cote JK, Godin G. Efficacy of interventions in improving adherence to antiretroviral therapy. *Int J STD AIDS.* 2005;16:225–343
51. Marlatt GA, Gordon JR. *Relapse Prevention Maintenance Strategies in the Treatment of Addictive Behaviors.* New York, NY: Guilford Press; 1985
52. Vasilaki EI, Hosier SG, Cox WM. The efficacy of motivational interviewing as a brief intervention for excessive drinking: a meta-analytic review. *Alcohol Alcohol.* 2006;41(3):328–335
53. Miller WR, Rollnick S. *Motivational Interviewing: Preparing People for Change.* 2nd ed. New York, NY: Guilford Press; 2002

54. Parsons JT, Rosof E, Punzalan JC, Di Maria L. Integration of motivational interviewing and cognitive behavioral therapy to improve HIV medication adherence and reduce substance use among HIV-positive men and women: results of a pilot project. *AIDS Patient Care STDS.* 2005;19(1):31-39
55. Golden MP, Herrold AJ, Orr DP. An approach to prevention of recurrent diabetic ketoacidosis in the pediatric population. *J Pediatr.* 1985;107(2):195-200
56. Rotherum-Borus MJ, Murphy DA, Coleman CL, Risk acts, health care, and medical adherence among HIV+ youths in care over time. *AIDS Behav.* 1997;1(1):43-52
57. Belzer ME, Fuchs DN, Luftman GS, Tucker DJ. Antiretroviral adherence issues among HIV-positive adolescents and young adults. *J Adolesc Health.* 1999;25(5):316-319
58. Wilson CM, Houser J, Partlow C, et al. The REACH (Reaching for Excellence in Adolescent Care and Health) Project: study design, methods, and population. *J Adolesc Health.* 2001;29(suppl 3):8-18
59. Flynn PM, Rudy BJ, Douglas SD, et al. Virologic and immunologic outcomes after 24 weeks in HIV type 1-infected adolescents receiving highly active antiretroviral therapy. *J Infect Dis.* 2004;190(2):271-279
60. Stilley CS, Lawrence K, Bender A, Olshansky E, Webber SA, Dew MA. Maturity and adherence in adolescent and young adult heart recipients. *Pediatr Transplant.* 2006;10(3):323-330
61. Fish L, Lung CL; Antileukotriene Working Group. Adherence to asthma therapy. *Ann Allergy Asthma Immunol.* 2001;86(6 suppl 1):24-30
62. Moos MK, Bartholomew NE, Lohr KN. Counseling in the clinical setting to prevent unintended pregnancy: an evidence-based research agenda. *Contraception.* 2003;67(2):115-132
63. Baker SA, Thalberg SP, Morrison DM. Parents' behavioral norms as predictors of adolescent sexual activity and contraceptive use. *Adolescence.* 1988;23(90):265-282
64. Jaccard J, Dittus PJ, Gordon VV. Maternal correlates of adolescent sexual and contraceptive behavior. *Fam Plann Perspect.*1996;28:159-165, 185
65. Glasgow AM, Weissberg-Benchell J, Tynan WD, et al. Readmission of children with diabetes mellitus to a children's hospital. *Pediatrics.* 1991;88(1):98-104
66. Iannotti RJ, Schneider S, Nansel TR, et al. Self-efficacy, outcome expectations, and diabetes self-management in adolescents with type 1 diabetes. *J Dev Behav Pediatr.* 2006;27(2):98-105
67. Ellis DA, Frey MA, Naar-King S, Templin T, Cunningham P, Cakan N. Use of multisystemic therapy to improve regimen adherence among adolescents with type 1 diabetes in chronic poor metabolic control: a randomized controlled trial. *Diabetes Care.* 2005;28(7):1604-1610
68. Alemzadeh R, Ellis J, Calhoun M, Kichler J. Predictors of metabolic control at one year in a population of pediatric patients with type 2 diabetes mellitus: a retrospective study. *J Pediatr Endocrinol Metab.* 2006;19(9):1141-1149

Communicating With Teens Who Are Living With Cancer

Olle Jane Z. Sahler, MD[a]*, Lauren Spiker, MEd[b]

[a]Departments of Pediatrics, Psychiatry, Medical Humanities, and Oncology, University of Rochester School of Medicine and Dentistry, and Division of Pediatric Hematology/Oncology, Golisano Children's Hospital at Strong, 601 Elmwood Avenue, Box 777, Rochester, NY 14642-8777, USA

[b]Melissa's Living Legacy Teen Cancer Foundation, 3111 Winton Road South, Rochester, NY 14623, USA

In April 1998, Melissa was a typical high school senior preparing for the senior ball, graduation, and life's many opportunities when she was diagnosed with myelodysplastic syndrome, a rare bone marrow malignancy. She had just been accepted to the University of Pennsylvania, where she had planned to pursue a career in advanced-practice nursing. Melissa died on June 22, 2000, at the age of 19 after living with cancer for 2 years. Melissa's and her family's experiences are recounted in the vignettes written by her mother, Lauren Spiker, that appear throughout this article.

In 2001, the Institute of Medicine published a blueprint for improving the quality of health care entitled *Crossing the Quality Chasm*.[1] After exhaustive research and extensive hearings, the Institute of Medicine concluded that the key strategy for improving the quality of health care is to practice patient-centered care, or care that is responsive to patient needs on the basis of mutual respect and shared decision-making. Although touted as a new paradigm, most people would call this good old-fashioned medicine. Others would remind us that there are both art and science to medicine, and the art of medicine is being a doctor ("one skilled . . . in the healing arts"[2]). Regrettably, in shedding our Norman Rockwellian image as kindly but woefully behind-the-times country doctors, we also shed some of the humanness that allowed us to recognize our inherent susceptibility to fallibility, emotional attachment, and distress over loss for ourselves and others. Virtually all that we will discuss in the next few pages stems from these human feelings that, we argue, are essential for the practice of good medicine.

---

*Corresponding author.
E-mail address: oj_sahler@urmc.rochester.edu (O. J. Z. Sahler).

Copyright © 2008 American Academy of Pediatrics. All rights reserved. ISSN 1934-4287

Unfortunately, they also lead to feelings of inadequacy, professional failure, and helplessness—feelings that physicians have apparently absorbed by osmosis as part of the "hidden curriculum."[3] Because no one will admit to actually teaching these hidden curricula to us, these feelings must have been modeled by teachers who had forgotten that although a doctor's mission is to cure often—indeed, as often as possible—his/her greater mission is to always care, and there is no failure in caring.

ROLE OF THE PRIMARY CARE PHYSICIAN

> April 3, 1998, 8:30 AM: I was working in my home office, sipping my third cup of coffee, when the telephone rang—just a normal morning, probably a client. It was Melissa's pediatrician.
>
> "Don't worry," he said. "We don't think it's anything life-threatening like leukemia but... you must get Melissa to the hospital immediately. Take her to the pediatric oncology clinic. They know you're coming."
>
> My heart stopped beating. In the space of a minute, the ordered life I had so carefully crafted had been shattered with a word: leukemia. Just a month before, when Melissa saw the pediatrician for her annual physical, her hemoglobin level had been a little low. "Probably just a bit iron deficient," he had said, "not uncommon for girls her age. Daily iron pills for a month should do the trick." A new red flag was raised at the follow-up appointment. "It's probably only mononucleosis or some virus that's going around," he said as he reported an even lower hemoglobin level. "Let's get some blood work, just to be safe." In just 2 days, we had gone from common teenage "mono" to cancer. This just couldn't be real.
>
> Melissa never saw her pediatrician again—no follow-up calls, no visits in the hospital, only a condolence call after she died. Thankfully, we were cared for by a competent, compassionate oncology team on whom we relied for all our needs. I knew the oncologist was keeping Melissa's pediatrician informed, and I often wondered, "Doesn't he even care?"

In 1999, Forest et al[4] investigated how and why pediatricians refer patients for specialty care. They found that in 75% of cases, the referral was for advice on diagnosis or treatment that the primary care physician would perform. The most common condition for which consultation was requested was otitis media, something seen a dozen times a week in office practice. In the remaining 25% of cases, either the specialist was asked to manage the condition by providing technical expertise (eg, surgery) or the specialist was asked to manage the condition. In the United States, there are ~50 000 pediatricians who provide primary care and ~90 000 family practitioners, many, if not all, of whom care for child or adolescent patients. Typically, 10 000 cases of childhood cancer are diagnosed each year. Thus, on average, a given pediatrician is likely to diagnose a child with cancer less than once every 10 years. Given the rapid advances in diagnosis and treatment, almost all child patients with cancer are cared for in 1 of the 200 specially designated childhood cancer centers in the country. In very rural areas, the primary care physician may administer chemotherapy according to protocol, but the number of such cases is quite small. Compared with caring for a patient with otitis, what, then, is the role of the primary pediatrician in caring for a patient such as Melissa?

Information Giving

> We were quickly escorted to the inner sanctum of the clinic. The attending physician introduced himself and the pediatric resident who was shadowing him. We later learned that his area of expertise was research, perhaps explaining why he launched head-on into a complicated explanation of Melissa's blood counts: white blood cell count, hematocrit, platelets, reticulocyte count, neutrophils, young cells, mature cells, antibodies, differentials, anemia, leukopenia, thrombocytopenia, pancytopenia . . ..
>
> "Stop! Wait!" I yelled out loud (or in my head, I don't know). "Just tell us what we need to do next. Just tell us the next step."
>
> In time, I would become extremely proficient in the use of medical terminology, able to banter with the best, but in those first frightening moments we just needed a reassuring voice, simple explanations with words no longer than 3 syllables, time between thoughts to process the reality, and a comforting hand extended in partnership. There would be time for the science later. Melissa said not a word through all of this. I know she was scared. So was I.
>
> More blood work was necessary. "Lab results are discouraging; all indicators are lower than 2 days ago. We need to do a bone marrow biopsy. Let's set up a time for you to meet the head of our bone marrow transplant team. How are you doing? I know this is a lot all at once. We don't really know; red blood cells are breaking down, and new ones are being produced faster than normal. Maybe you're losing blood somewhere, but your white blood cell count is also down, which seems consistent with myelodysplastic syndrome, a bone marrow infiltration process that is extremely rare, especially in young people. Sometimes it's called preleukemia or smoldering leukemia; a bone marrow biopsy will confirm the diagnosis. See Dr B. at 10:00 on Tuesday, April 7th. Try to have a good weekend."
>
> We were standing in the small lounge outside the treatment area. Every word, every sentence ran into the next. I'm not sure I looked at his face,

and I don't know if he looked at ours; I do know I looked at Melissa's, and my heart tore in two, wishing I could take her place. It was Friday afternoon—quiet. I don't remember any other patients. I don't remember what the weather was like. I don't remember what she wore—jeans, probably. I don't remember saying good-bye.

What I do remember is leaving the clinic and life as we knew it. Whatever her disease was, it was not trivial. Although I, like many parents, try to prepare for the worst-case scenario, no disaster fantasy can match the emotional punch of hearing that your child has cancer.

Looking back, I wish that our pediatrician had prepared us for all of this. Although he could not be sure of the diagnosis until after all the studies were performed, I wish that he had said he would be available to talk to us. Even though we were well informed and didn't feel the need to call him, I wish he had called us at least once.

How bad news is presented affects understanding,[5] satisfaction,[6,7] degree of hopefulness,[8] and psychological adjustment.[9–11] Effective communication provides listeners with the information they need in a form that they can easily comprehend.[12] Accomplishing this task requires that the transmitter of the information determine what is most worth saying and that the receiver of the information integrate the message into his or her own cognitive processes and life experience. In this case, information about an unfamiliar diagnosis is often fragmentary at best. The lack of background knowledge is problematic and complicated further by the impact that bad news has on our ability to absorb distressing information. Although potentially destructive in the long term, early on, cognitive processes such as denial serve the useful function of limiting the rate and extent of knowledge integration and, thus, mitigate the degree of emotional overload that assaults the listener. As Melissa's mother explained, no matter how "prepared" you believe you are, nothing really prepares you for hearing that your child has cancer.

Why, similar to the oncologist in this vignette, do doctors talk too much when giving bad news? In this case, the most likely reason for the physician's long recital of apparently extraneous information is twofold: (1) to build up personal readiness to use the word "cancer" to cope with the emotional outpouring that might come from the family, although there is little evidence that receiving unfavorable medical information inevitability causes psychological harm,[13,14] and (2) in the hope that by using words that the patient and family might know in other contexts (eg, malignancy, tumor) they will be the ones to use the word "cancer" first (ie, it is much easier to respond "yes" to "You mean my daughter has cancer?") or that the family may never need to have the word spoken (whatever the disease, be it muscular dystrophy, diabetes, or Crohn disease) to understand what is being said. Studies have shown that the bearer of bad news frequently is anxious, feels some responsibility for the news, and fears being seen negatively by the people to whom the news is brought. These stresses magnify the innate reluctance to deliver bad news that is inherent in all of us.[15]

Why, like the primary care physician in this vignette, might a doctor relinquish all contact? The literature on what to do in this circumstance is sparse. However, we can use the primary physician's role after the death of a child as an analogy. After all, some hope, dream, or expectation for the child has just died, and the family is suffering. Wessel[16] reminded us that the primary physician has a potentially enormous role to play as a person who may have known the child for a long time. The time of diagnosis is an opportunity to visit at the hospital or home or to communicate by telephone or e-mail that he or she cares and wishes to be helpful and supportive. Will the physician be able to answer all the family's questions? No. However, the visit is not about answering questions, it is about telling them that he/she know what has happened, we know that this is a very trying time, and if there is any way we can help by, for example, talking with the other children in the family, he/she is ready to do it. Or, if siblings come to the office for an acute illness or routine care, the doctor can acknowledge that this is a tough time for everyone in the family, including them, and offer to answer questions or just give a pat on the back. Or, just send a card or e-mail message: "I saw an article about your school in the newspaper yesterday and immediately wondered how you're doing. Please remember that I'm thinking of you all. Don't hesitate to call if I can be of help." Or, "Dr B. called me to tell me that it looks like you'll need a transplant. I know this isn't news that you wanted to hear, but I know you're in good hands. Please remember that I'm always hoping for the best for you." Melissa's illness lasted for ~2 years. Four or 5 messages or calls would have reassured the family that her pediatrician cared.

> Tuesday finally came after a long weekend of researching myelodysplasia on the Internet. Terminology that had been foreign just days before was now part of our daily conversation. We were armed with information and questions. Melissa had her own set of concerns, including when she could return to swim practice.
>
> We spent some time exchanging pleasantries with Dr B. (trying to build rapport), for which Melissa had little patience on this tense day. She was very good at getting right to business. I knew he was struggling, grappling for just the right words to explain the enormous challenges that faced this beautiful young girl whom he had just met.
>
> I remember feeling impatient, too, as he repeated much of what we had heard the previous Friday. Dr B. talked a little too much when giving us difficult news. I always thought it was a coping strategy he used to keep himself from getting emotionally involved, although we were told later that Melissa "had gotten to him." It was easier to keep talking than

to endure the deafening silence. I bombarded him with questions. I clearly recall him saying more than once, "This probably won't make much sense right now" as he proceeded to answer every question. I never felt dismissed or hurried, but in all the words spoken, there were 2 words Dr B. never uttered: "cancer" and "dying."

Because physicians are human beings who chose medicine to save life, not destroy it, telling bad news can be thought of as the destruction of a safe, even-keeled existence and a particularly devastating blow to an adolescent whose life is just unfolding. No physician takes pride in doing that. Fortunately, some realize that breaking down can be followed by building up, and it is here that the art of medicine provides a return to wholeness through caring. It is also useful to remember that although bad news may sadden the patient, it may be essential for realistically planning for the future and achieving certain goals that can ease existential pain.

What is also often forgotten is that all the words surrounding, in this case, the "C" word fall on deaf ears, even if the patient's face, mouth, and head move in ways that mimic understanding. Even if questions are asked that are sensible and appropriate, even if comforting hands on shoulders or hugs are exchanged, as Melissa's mother tells us, the reality is beyond any expectation. Every fiber of the collective family's being prays that what has just transpired is, indeed, only a dream or, at the very least, not as bad as it seems. How often do physicians feel frustration, annoyance, and self-righteousness when they hear from families—or, worse yet, other health care providers in what seem to be accusatory tones—that they never told the patient "X" when, in fact, they said it not once but twice or even more?

Again, thinking back to the shock and denial the adolescent and family are experiencing, it becomes clear that repetition is critical to understanding. At the point at which they recognize that they do not have particular information, they are more likely to finally hear what has already been said. Simply saying, "I mentioned this before, but perhaps I said it too quickly," makes the point that you have not been delinquent and share the responsibility for active listening between physician and family. Remember that they are dealing with a massive blow to their very being; the physician's own bruised ego is hardly comparable. Encounters like this, however difficult, are the building blocks of strong partnerships from which effective communication patterns will develop.

As pointed out by the SIOP Working Committee on Psychosocial Issues in Pediatric Oncology,[17] "it should be understood that communication is a continuing process, not a single event. It may take parents and children several meetings and conversations with physicians before they are fully aware of the implications of [the disease and treatment]." Furthermore, "[c]ommunication is a continual two-way process over time. A healthy and open level of communication from the very beginning makes continued conversation less burdensome and more helpful when later treatment complexities arise."[18] These are among the most important take-away points of the entire document, whether talking about cancer or some other problem: start conversing early and reiterate frequently. Failure of the family to understand is expected. Failure on our part to repeat the information is inexcusable.

Building Rapport

> Each month, a new attending physician took the lead in directing Melissa's care. It seemed that as soon as we had established a comfortable rapport we needed to shift gears and "break in" a new doctor. Connecting with teenagers is not always easy, and the standard first line "So, tell me what brought you here" sure doesn't help. More than once, both my daughter and I wanted to say, "Is there something in the chart you don't understand?" One particular introduction was different from the rest, however. When Dr C. met Melissa for the first time, he earned her immediate respect, not because he wore a white coat but because he took just 2 minutes to comment on her T-shirt's logo, which he recognized. She never forgot that simple gesture, which made her feel like a valued individual and not "the leukemia in room 238."

What is rapport? Wikipedia (http://en.wikipedia.org/wiki/Main_Page) defines it as one of the most important features or characteristics of unconscious human interaction. It is commonality of perspective, being "in sync," being on the same wavelength as the person with whom you are interacting. Why would it be important for a physician to establish rapport with a patient and family? One particular reason is to ensure that everyone is in agreement regarding the extent and duration of treatment, the potential adverse effects and their management, and their appraisal of the anticipated benefits, that is, that they are in agreement that they are forming a partnership. Forming a partnership, however, means recognizing that the partners have equal status, cooperate closely, and recognize joint rights and responsibilities. The burden of maintaining the partnership falls on all parties, who must be truthful, conscientious, and willing to honestly consider others' points of view. Rapport begins by acknowledging the value of the other person. In the vignette, the simple gesture of noticing that something is important enough to the patient to wear it as an emblem tacitly states that you recognize that the patient has many personal dimensions that existed before the cancer and that will live outside and beyond the cancer. For the physician and patient, the major connection between them is the disease and its treatment, but both have other likes, dislikes, stresses, and passions that add depth to the decisions that each will make regarding providing and accepting health care. Knowing about these "peripheral" issues deepens the type of relationship that is essential for the best care to take place. It is important to note that rapport can take place without "rap"; there is no need for the physician to feel compelled to adopt the jargon *du jour* to gain the trust and, most importantly, respect of the teenaged patient. In fact, recognizing that there is a difference between you and the patient with regard to life experience and expertise is comforting to teens. They want to feel that they are in good hands.

In a study of Australian teens and young adults, the health care professional's ability to listen, show genuine concern, demonstrate expertise, and be honest versus having an impersonal manner, using technical jargon, being hasty, and falling into the generation gap facilitated communication between them and their doctor.[19]

Bridging the generation gap with adolescents is critical for establishing rapport and building trust. Everything from fashion to lifestyle and language differences can create barriers between a physician and adolescent patients and impede effective communication. Rapid advances in technology are changing the way in which teens both receive and transmit information, thereby potentially further widening the gap. Authors of the 2005 Pew Internet & American Life Project[20] surveyed a random sample of 1100 parent-child pairs to better understand the communication style of adolescents. The investigators found that 87% of US teens use the Internet, and 51% of those go online daily. This equates to ~11 million teens using the Internet every day. By contrast, only 66% of adults are Internet users.

Adolescents surf the Internet to play games, get news, make purchases, and access health care information. The highest percentage of teen Internet activity centers around connecting with others: 89% of teen Internet users use e-mail, and the vast majority prefer instant messaging as their mode of communication. In addition, almost 50% of all teenagers in the United States own a cell phone, many with text-messaging capability and Internet connectivity. An entirely new language convention, entirely foreign to most adults, has been developed to facilitate on-line communication.[21]

So, what is the relevance of technology to health care professionals who hope to establish rapport with their teen patients? It is simply to understand the tools as common ground and perhaps use them for improved delivery of care. Using cancer as an example, the Web site Teens Living With Cancer (www.teenslivingwithcancer.org) is a comprehensive site cosponsored by Melissa's Living Legacy Teen Cancer Foundation and the Children's Oncology Group, a National Cancer Institute-supported research cooperative of more than 250 pediatric oncology hospitals worldwide. The site, which averages more than 90 000 hits per week with very active message boards and interactive functionality, is designed specifically for teens and uses familiar language and concepts. Medical information is reviewed by a medical editorial board to ensure accuracy, but all the design features are monitored by a teen advisory council that ensures the "coolness" factor.

Health care professionals can glean important perspective from visiting a site like this, reviewing how the material is presented, and reading the anonymous but candid message boards. To ensure understanding of treatment options and offer additional psychosocial support, physicians can recommend such a reliable site to reinforce what has been discussed in the hospital or office. A 2003 study that was undertaken by the University of Michigan Health System investigated how teenagers search the Internet for health information. Their findings revealed that misspelled words, ambiguous search terms, and an imprecise approach to scanning a Web site often prevent young people from finding appropriate information. Given the high percentage of teens who use the Internet regularly (many of whom are seeking health care information) and the large body of inaccurate and misleading information on the Web, it is essential that physicians direct their teenaged patients to accurate and safe sites.

If rapport, as stated earlier, is being in sync with another person and having a common perspective, it seems reasonable that all opportunities to understand the lifestyle of teenaged patients should be explored, even if it requires stretching outside adult comfort zones. Seeing what draws them to a Web site about cancer (or any disease) provides vital information about how the diagnosis and its treatment should be presented to enhance understanding and long-term commitment to therapy. One would think that treatment compliance would be excellent among teens with a life-threatening illness such as cancer. However, it is known that compliance is actually poor among adults,[22–25] let alone teens,[26,27] despite the fact that treatment currently is given with the intent to cure not merely to palliate. We also know that, among pediatric patients, adolescents are less compliant than younger patients and need to be involved more fully in the process of informed consent regarding their own treatment.[28]

Common reasons for refusal, noncompliance, and abandonment of therapy include pain/discomfort (eg, chemotherapy-induced nausea), fear of disfigurement (alopecia, amputation), misunderstanding and uncertainty about the merits of a given treatment, and poor understanding of the seriousness of the illness. Conflicts between adolescents and their parents over who "owns" the disease become magnified instances of typical teen-parent disagreements. It is unfortunate that, for whatever reason, noncompliance can literally mean the difference between life and death.

EMPOWERMENT

> After much testing and second opinions by bone marrow experts across the country, Melissa's diagnosis was finally confirmed: myelodysplasia, type RAEB-t (refractory anemia with excess blasts in transformation). Despite not being able to find a well-matched donor, we began planning for a bone marrow transplant began. Throughout all the months of uncertainty, Melissa continued her life as a normal teen. She

kept attending school, took 5 advanced-placement examinations, went to her senior ball, swam in the annual synchronized-swim show, and graduated fourth in her class of 380 students. One event remained on her checklist: a long-awaited trip to Germany with a friend.

From a scheduling perspective, Melissa's trip did not interfere with the transplant. It would be late July at the earliest before all systems would be ready, but my steadfast opinion about taking this trip was, "No way!" What if she got sick thousands of miles away? What if she needed a blood transfusion? How could she carry her luggage? What if she needed me and I couldn't be there? Melissa, however, was determined to go. I remember asking Dr B. his advice and will never forget his sober response: "You have to let her go. There are no guarantees." To Melissa, he simply said, "Have a great time! We'll get started when you get home."

So, we packed. Alongside her other essentials were blood vials, lab orders, and an extensive medical history with contact information for a doctor in Berlin, just in case. Looking back, I have no doubt that this trip fortified Melissa for the road ahead. I remain ever grateful that Dr B. supported her need for independence and adventure.

In their study of teens with chronic illness, Britto et al[29] asked 155 patients aged 11 to 19 years to list and then prioritize their health care preferences and expectations. Physician honesty, attention to patient pain, and expertise ranked highest with regard to medical care. The highest-rated items with regard to physician communication were explaining things so they, rather than just their parents, could understand, speaking with them privately and confidentially, and telling them about their treatment first.

These responses clearly highlight the major paradoxes of the chronically ill adolescent: (1) having emerging capabilities in the face of diminishing possibilities and (2) lacking legal authority to make binding medical decisions despite meeting the functional criteria for having the competence to do so (full awareness of the consequences of agreeing or disagreeing to undergo particular treatments).[30]

Most societies are in agreement that at the age of majority (typically 18 years), an adolescent has the right to make all medical care decisions for himself or herself. Most institutions work hard to help the family come to consensus if disagreement exists, but the right of the competent older adolescent to make final decisions regarding care is indisputable. The answers to the questions raised by Britto et al and the age range of the youth who participated in their study (mean age: 15.5 years) showed that the desire for full information, preferably before it is given to parents, begins in early to midadolescence. The struggle the family undergoes is permitting the patient to increase his or her authority for self-determination at the same time that he or she is becoming increasingly dependent on the family for care in all other aspects of life.

SHARED DECISION-MAKING

> It soon became apparent to Melissa's team that she was very capable of managing her own self-care. One of the first tasks she insisted on doing herself was changing the daily dressing on her central line. She mastered the fine art of donning sterilized gloves much more readily than I. As a prospective nursing student, she learned not only how to perform her own granulocyte colony-stimulating factor injections but also gave the nurses in clinic their influenza shots that fall. Consequently, Melissa was always included in pertinent discussions about her treatment and was treated as an equal player when it came to information sharing and negotiating hospital schedules. Although she was smart enough to not take unnecessary risks, she advocated for herself extremely well. I remember the weekend she wanted to visit her boyfriend at college. Being fully aware of what sometimes happens in college dorm rooms, I was more nervous than usual at the thought of Melissa being away with a boy. A sensitive but candid "lecture" about the dangers of having sex while undergoing cancer treatment was very welcomed when delivered by her nurse practitioner without me present. I remember feeling relieved, and impressed, with the nurse's straightforward and honest communication style.

With cognitive functioning in the formal operational stage, teens show an intellectual capacity to reason, generalize beyond personal experience, deal with abstract ideas, and hypothesize or predict potential consequences of actions. Apart from inexperience, most individuals aged 14 years and older have the same capacities to process information as adults.[31] Bibace and Walsh[32] found that more than 40% of 11-year-old children understood that disease has a physiologic basis. Thus, children begin to understand disease processes around the age of 11 and demonstrate the competence to make treatment decisions by the age of 14.

Virtually all states recognize the emancipated minor (ie, married or living independently without parental financial support) as a person who is able to make his or her own health care decisions. The concept of the mature minor (an individual who is capable of fully appreciating the nature and consequences of a particular treatment), however, is not recognized in all states, although it is part of Canadian law.[33] The concept of the mature minor is a higher standard than that of the emancipated minor, because it demands specific knowledge and understanding, rather than mere circumstances, to grant decision-making rights.

> It had been 6 weeks since Dr B. conveyed the good news that Melissa was in remission. Arduous chemotherapy was replaced by weekly

blood draws and a return to a new normalcy, including a planned trip to New York City with 4 friends. All was once again right with the world until we received the latest lab results. Melissa's counts were down. When asked what could have caused the drop, the nurse practitioner replied, "Maybe just a virus"—a virus, again. How many times had we heard that? Lab results 2 weeks later confirmed what we hadn't dared to consciously think about: it wasn't a virus, and we knew it wouldn't be. But Dr B. couldn't say the word: "relapse." He didn't have to.

Instead, he talked about next steps and suggested another bone marrow biopsy just to be sure. If the results confirmed his suspicion, Melissa would need to start chemo immediately and begin preparing for a bone marrow transplant. We listened without interruption. I asked mostly logistic questions: "Who? What? Where?" I don't remember what my husband said, but I'll never forget Melissa's simple, direct question: "Can we wait until Monday?" She had plans that weekend in New York City. Dr B. said, "Yes."

Part of me wanted her to stay home, away from the dirty subways and questionable street life of New York City, safely sanitized and protected from the world she craved to experience. My better, but more frightened, side let her go.

In adolescent decision-making, the "proportionality" of a decision (eg, the elective amputation of a limb with possibly metastatic disease versus the withdrawing of life-sustaining treatment) may be considered.[34] Proportionality refers to a "sliding scale" of competency: the more important or serious the outcome, the higher the level of competency that should be required to make that decision. According to the American Academy of Pediatrics, "physicians and parents should give great weight to clearly expressed views of child patients regarding [life-sustaining medical treatment], regardless of the legal particulars."[35] Similarly, the Society for Adolescent Medicine has stated that an adolescent should have a major decision-making role in agreeing to participate, for example, in the research process.[36] Typically, this caveat has been considered to be particularly true if the research project represented a phase I or even phase II trial. Although neither the American Academy of Pediatrics nor the Society for Adolescent Medicine endorses sole decision-making by the pediatric patient, the shift from "great weight" being given to children's opinions to "major" decision-making by adolescents reflects the growing influence of the child's wishes as he or she matures. Although most formal discussion of the capacity of pediatric patients to make informed decisions has centered on life-sustaining treatments and research participation, proponents of greater child-patient participation in decision-making have suggested that all clinical situations be opened for discussion at the policy-making level.[31]

Optimally, the adolescent does participate in all health care decisions, including those that concern life-sustaining medical treatment, with the health care team and parents in a supportive environment. Occasionally, parents and teens will disagree. Under this circumstance, all parties should receive accurate information on prognosis, treatment options, and clinical course with and without treatment. The physician should assess an adolescent's ability to comprehend and reflect on the choices available,to balance risks and benefits, and to understand the implications of his or her decisions. When an adolescent has the capacity to make competent health care decisions, the ethical physician should allow the adolescent the right to exercise his or her autonomy.[31]

END OF LIFE

> There is "bad news" and "really bad news." Having to tell a vibrant, beautiful teenager that she is going to die is never easy. Even the most effective communicators find it difficult to balance professional obligation and personal emotion. Melissa was fortunate to have a medical team that not only took care of her medical condition but truly cared about her as a person. After 2 years of treatment, she had come to trust her primary oncologist and nurse practitioner implicitly. We got very good at "reading" faces and always knew the "look" of bad news. There are times, however, when words are necessary if, for nothing else, to maintain consistency and clarity, especially when emotions cloud the picture. I remember waiting for the results of a bone marrow biopsy after Melissa's second relapse, bone marrow transplant, and treatment with an experimental drug. We all knew the look, but the words just didn't match. "The results show that the medicines didn't work like we'd hoped they would," said Dr B. We all knew what he meant but couldn't say—Melissa was going to die. Maybe he felt a failure for not being able to save her life, or maybe he was just sad like the rest of us, but it would have helped to put a name on the elephant in the room. We wouldn't have been angry with him and certainly wouldn't have blamed him. Of course, we still would have cried, but at least we could have talked about how to walk around the beast in a way that made sense for everyone, especially Melissa, who had very definite opinions about how she wanted to live—and die.
>
> Melissa made her final decision to stop all treatment. She had come to accept that her time on Earth was very limited. She knew how sick chemotherapy would make her feel and opted for quality of life versus quantity. An entry in her journal reads, "I don't feel as if I'm giving up just because I'm opting for no treatment. All other options are noncurative ... may slow the process and give me another week? Another month? But at what cost to me, I ask? I'm not giving up. I fought hard

> for 2 years. I survived those years—with pride. And I did a lot. Now it is time. It is the next step in the plan."

In the 3 months until she died, Melissa never stopped living. She took a vacation with her family to the Grand Canyon, rode a hot air balloon over the Arizona desert, planted an herb garden, crocheted an afghan, and took a pottery class, all while writing poetry and prose in her journal. She said goodbye to her friends and family. She made plans for her death and burial and donating her body for medical study.

Communication with patients of any age who have moved to the stage of terminal illness is fraught with the complicated emotions of knowing that it is likely that the patient will die, soon. Trainees and experienced professionals alike report that the 1 question they fear the most is, "Am I going to die?" Most have gotten beyond, "Everybody dies sometime." Some temporize behind, "I don't know," which is hardly true because everybody dies sometime. Almost all have stopped saying, "Of course not!"

Although it is difficult to confront this issue directly, it is useful to recall the Britto et al study[29] in which adolescents listed physician honesty as their most important expectation. They need to know the truth and are generally capable of dealing with it. In fact, many teens who have experienced failed treatment, like Melissa, already have a sense that they will die as a result of their disease. So, what might the patient really be asking? The simplest way to discover what is most troubling is to respond with a request: "You've been thinking about it. Tell me what you've been thinking." Sometimes the answer is, "Who will take care of my dog?" or "Will it hurt?" or, most poignantly, "Will you forget me?" Being remembered for who they were and what they contributed to the world is one way in which adolescents, like all of us, ascribe meaning to their life and death.

> Just 3 nights before Melissa died, we talked late into the night. I told her how proud I was of her and how she had lived her life and thanked her for all she had taught me. In response, she asked a promise of me: "If you've learned anything from me through all of this, do something with it to make a difference—to make things better."

REFERENCES

1. Institute of Medicine. *Crossing the Quality Chasm: A New Health System for the 21st Century.* Washington, DC: National Academy Press; 2001
2. Mish FC. *Merriam-Webster's Collegiate Dictionary*, 10th ed. Springfield, MA: Merriam-Webster, Inc; 1994:341
3. Hafferty FW, Franks R. The hidden curriculum, ethics teaching, and the structure of medical education. *Acad Med.* 1994;69(11):861–871

4. Forrest CB, Glade GB, Baker AE, Bocian AB, Kang M, Starfield B. The pediatric primary-specialty care interface: how pediatricians refer children and adolescents to specialty care. *Arch Pediatr Adolesc Med.* 1999;153(7):705–714
5. Maynard DW. On "realization" in everyday life: the forecasting of bad news as a social relation. *Am Sociol Rev.* 1996;61(1):109–131
6. Ford S, Fallowfield L, Lewis S. Doctor-patient interaction in oncology. *Soc Sci Med.* 1996; 42(11):1511–1519
7. Butow PN, Dunn SM, Tattersall MH. Communication with cancer patients: does it matter? *J Palliat Care.* 1995;11(4):34–38
8. Sardell AN, Trierweiler SJ. Disclosing the cancer diagnosis: procedures that influence patient hopefulness. *Cancer.* 1993;72(11):3355–3365
9. Roberts CS, Cox CE, Reintgen DS, Baile WF, Gibertini M. Influence of physician communication on newly diagnosed breast patients' psychologic adjustment and decision-making. *Cancer.* 1994;74(1 suppl):336–341
10. Slavin LA, O'Malley JE, Koocher GP, Foster DJ. Communication of the cancer diagnosis to pediatric patients: impact on long-term adjustment. *Am J Psychiatry.* 1982;139(2):179–183
11. Last BF, van Veldhuizen AM. Information about diagnosis and prognosis related to anxiety and depression in children with cancer aged 8–16 years. *Eur J Cancer.* 1996;32A(2):290–294
12. Fischhoff B. Why (cancer) risk communication can be hard. *J Natl Cancer Inst Monogr.* 1999;25(25):7–13
13. Cassem NH, Stewart RS. Management and care of the dying patient. *Int J Psychiatry Med.* 1975;6(1–2):293–304
14. Pfeifer MP, Sidorov JE, Smith AC, Boero JF, Evans AT, Settle MB. The discussion of end-of-life medical care by primary care patients and physicians: a multicenter study using structured qualitative interviews. The EOL Study Group. *J Gen Intern Med.* 1994;9(2):82–88
15. Tesser A, Rosen S, Tesser M. On the reluctance to communicate undesirable messages (the MUM effect): a field study. *Psychol Rep.* 1971;29(2):651–654
16. Wessel MA. The primary physician and the death of a child in a specialized hospital setting. *Pediatrics.* 1983;71(3):443–445
17. Spinetta JJ, Masera G, Jankovic M, et al. Valid informed consent and participative decision-making in children with cancer and their parents: a report of the SIOP Working Committee on psychosocial issues in pediatric oncology. *Med Pediatr Oncol.* 2003;40(4):244–246
18. Masera G, Chesler MA, Jankovic M, et al. SIOP working committee on psychosocial issues in pediatric oncology: guidelines for communication of the diagnosis. *Med Pediatr Oncol.* 1997; 28(5):382–385
19. Dunsmore J, Quine S. Information, support, and decision-making needs and preferences of adolescents with cancer: implications for health professionals. *J Psychosoc Oncol.* 1995;13(4): 39–56
20. Lenhart A, Madden M, Hitlin P. Teens and technology: youth are leading the transition to a fully wired and mobile nation. Available at: www.pewinternet.org/pdfs/PIP_Teens_Tech_July2005web.pdf. Accessed December 31, 2007
21. Hansen DL, Derry HA, Resnick PJ, Richardson CR. Adolescents searching for health information on the internet: an observational study. *J Med Internet Res.* 2003;5(4):e25
22. Taylor SE, Lichtmann RR, Wood JV. Compliance with chemotherapy among breast cancer patients. *Health Psychol.* 1984;3(6):553–562
23. Lee YT. Adjuvant chemotherapy (CMF) for breast carcinoma: patient's compliance and total dose achieved. *Am J Clin Oncol.* 1983;6(1):25–30
24. Berger D, Braverman A, Sohn CK, Morrow M. Patient compliance with aggressive multimodal therapy in locally advanced breast cancer. *Cancer.* 1988;61(7):1453–1456
25. Richardson JL, Marks G, Johnson CA, et al. Path model of multidimensional compliance with cancer therapy. *Health Psychol.* 1987;6(3):183–207
26. Smith SD, Rosen D, Trueworthy RC, Lowman JT. A reliable method for evaluating drug compliance in children with cancer. *Cancer.* 1979;43(1):169–173

27. Tebbi CK, Cummings KM, Zevon MA, Smith L, Richards M, Mallon J. Compliance of pediatric and adolescent cancer patients. *Cancer*. 1986;58(5):1179–1184
28. Spinetta JJ, Masera G, Eden T, et al. Refusal, non-compliance, and abandonment of treatment in children and adolescents with cancer: a report of the SIOP Working Committee on Phychosocial Issues in Pediatric Oncology. *Med Pediatr Oncol*. 2002;38(2):114–117
29. Britto MT, DeVellis RF, Hornung RW, DeFriese GH, Atherton HD, Slap GB. Health care preferences and priorities of adolescents with chronic illnesses. *Pediatrics*. 2004;114(5):1272–1280
30. Freyer DR. Care of the dying adolescent: special considerations. *Pediatrics*. 2004;113(2):381–388
31. Doig C, Burgess E. Withholding life-sustaining treatment: are adolescents competent to make these decisions? *CMAJ*. 2000;162(11):1585–1588
32. Bibace R, Walsh ME. Development of children's concepts of illness. *Pediatrics*. 1980;66(6): 912–917
33. Rozovsky LE. *Children, Adolescents, and Consent: The Canadian Law of Consent to Treatment.* 2nd ed. Toronto, Ontario, Canada: Butterworths; 1997:61–75
34. Gaylin W. The competence of children: no longer all or none. *Hastings Cent Rep*. 1982;12:33–38
35. American Academy of Pediatrics, Committee on Bioethics. Guidelines on foregoing life-sustaining medical treatment. *Pediatrics*. 1994;93(3):532–536
36. Sigman G, Silber TJ, English A, Gans Epner JE. Confidential health care for adolescents: position paper of the Society for Adolescent Medicine. *J Adolesc Health*. 1997;21(6):408–415

Serological Diagnosis of Infectious Diseases in the Adolescent

Christopher M. Oberholzer, MD,
Melanie Wellington, MD, PhD*

Division of Pediatric Infectious Diseases, Department of Pediatrics, University of Rochester School of Medicine and Dentistry, 601 Elmwood Avenue, Rochester, NY 14642, USA

As adolescents begin to gain their independence, they engage in behaviors that can result in exposure to new infectious diseases. At particular risk are adolescents who engage in high-risk sexual encounters, which may result in infections such as hepatitis C (HCV) and HIV. In other instances, adolescents may be acquiring ubiquitous microorganisms that are typically asymptomatic early in childhood but can result in significant symptoms during adolescence, such as Epstein-Barr virus (EBV) and, on occasion, cytomegalovirus (CMV). Serological testing in symptomatic adolescents can be very useful as a means to diagnose these infections. Serological assays may also be useful screening tools for detecting asymptomatic disease in adolescents at high risk.

The majority of serological assays are based on detecting host antibody responses to infection. After exposure to an infecting agent, an individual will typically mount an initial antibody response that is lower in specificity but can be produced relatively quickly. This response is typically composed of immunoglobulin M (IgM) antibodies. As the exposure or infection continues, antibody responses become more specialized. IgG antibodies that are highly specific with greater affinity for the antigenic structure of the infecting microorganism are produced.

Thus, over the course of an infection, antibody responses change from the initial IgM to the more specific IgG. An understanding of this process is useful for the clinician, because it facilitates detection of exposure, ongoing infection, and/or immunity to pathogens. The time course involved in the emergence of IgG antibodies is important in helping patients understand their symptoms and the expectations for resolution of disease. In some instances, antibody testing alone is not sufficient for accurate diagnosis. In these cases, the use of supplemental tests such as polymerase chain reaction (PCR) is required.

*Corresponding author.
E-mail address: melanie_wellington@urmc.rochester.edu (M. Wellington).

Adolescents are a unique group of pediatric patients with behaviors that put them at increased risk for developing infectious diseases such as mononucleosis and hepatitis. Serology is the mainstay of diagnosis for many of these infections. Serological methods can be extremely useful when used properly. In this article we review a number of serological tests and their interpretations as they apply to some important infectious conditions that are frequently encountered by adolescent patients.

INFECTIOUS MONONUCLEOSIS

The infectious disease most commonly associated with adolescence is infectious mononucleosis. The ailment classically presents as a febrile illness accompanied by malaise or fatigue, pharyngitis, and generalized lymphadenopathy. Some patients also have a rash, hepatomegaly, and/or splenomegaly. The most common pathogen responsible is EBV. Less frequently, mononucleosis can be caused by CMV, HIV, adenovirus, hepatitis A, and toxoplasmosis.

EBV is a ubiquitous virus that has a high seroprevalence in adults, ranging up to 90% to 95% in developed countries. In developing nations, most children are infected asymptomatically with EBV by 3 years of age.[1] In areas of higher socioeconomic status, more children encounter the virus for the first time as adolescents. When infection with EBV occurs during adolescence or young adulthood, it causes infectious mononucleosis 35% to 50% of the time.[2]

Patients with symptoms of infectious mononucleosis should be evaluated in a stepwise manner that begins with the commonly available heterophile antibody test or "monospot." Formal serological testing for EBV and CMV should be reserved for those adolescents who have a negative heterophile antibody test result and severe symptoms, especially those who are missing significant time from school and other activities.

The heterophile antibody assay measures the ability of the patient's nonspecific IgM antibodies to agglutinate the red blood cells of nonhuman species such as horses or sheep. Heterophile antibodies are usually detectable by the first 2 weeks of infection with EBV mononucleosis and gradually disappear over the following 6 months. False-negative test results are more likely to occur in the first week of symptoms. Heterophile antibody tests are most useful in children who are >10 years of age with classic symptoms of acute infectious mononucleosis. If the test result is positive in an appropriate clinical situation, no additional testing is necessary. The sensitivity and specificity of this test are 85% and 97%, respectively, in children >4 years of age.[3] False-negative results may be obtained in 10% to 15% of patients, primarily in children <10 years of age.[2] The rapid test that is used most commonly in modern clinical laboratories is based on the heterophile assay; however, it uses a solid-phase technology in which a color reaction is visible on the readout (often in the form of a "+" or "−" symbol).

This technique provides a more rapid methodology that is coupled with slightly higher sensitivity and specificity than the original heterophile antibody test.[4] The monospot test is the most common form of initial screening test in clinical laboratories.

Specific serological testing for EBV is useful for confirming the diagnosis in symptomatic adolescents when heterophile antibody test results are negative or in complex clinical situations. During the first several weeks of EBV infection, IgM antibody against the viral capsid antigen (IgM-VCA), the corresponding IgG antibody (IgG-VCA), and antibodies against early antigen (EA, also called IgG-EA) are usually elevated (Fig 1). The rise of both IgM and IgG antibodies early in the disease process can make the interpretation of these tests difficult when testing is performed early. IgM-VCA can be detected in the first few weeks and usually disappears within 3 months.[5] The presence of IgM-VCA antibody is usually adequate for the diagnosis of acute disease caused by EBV. IgG-VCA also can be detected in the first few weeks of infection, but is usually present for life. EA antibody titers peak during convalescence and are typically detectable for several months after infection. However, up to 20% of healthy individuals have detectable levels of EA antibodies for years after infection.[2] Antibodies to EBV-determined nuclear antigen (EBNA, also called IgG-NA) can be found several months into infection/convalescence and are present for life. If IgM-VCA antibody is present with antibodies to EBNA, infection in the preceding 4 to 6

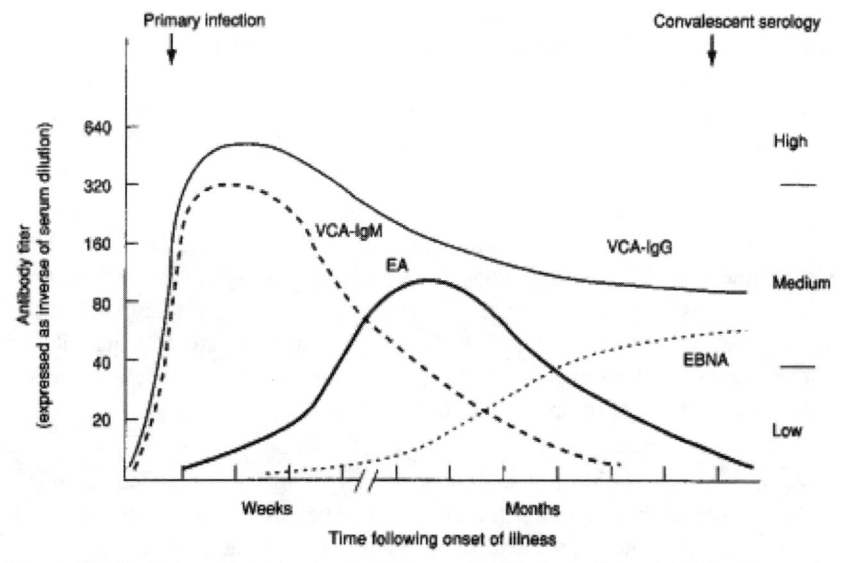

Fig 1. Idealized time course for the development of antibody to different EBV antigens after primary infection with the virus. EA: antibody against early antigen; EBNA: antibody against EBV-determined nuclear antigen. (Reproduced with permission from Long SS. *Principles and Practice of Pediatric Infectious Diseases*. 2nd ed. Philadelphia, PA: Churchill Livingstone, an imprint of Elsevier; 2003: 1062.).

months is most likely. Detection of antibodies to EBNA in the absence of IgM-VCA indicates a past infection.

As with other human herpes viruses, EBV is never completely eradicated but, instead, persists in a latent form that is usually held in check by normal cell-mediated immunity. In very few patients, typically those who for various reasons are immunocompromised, such as in those receiving solid organ or bone marrow transplants, EBV can reactivate. Reactivation of EBV is unlikely to lead to significant clinical illness in an immunocompetent individual. If the syndrome of infectious mononucleosis occurs in an individual who has a history of a previous episode of mononucleosis, it is likely that the episodes were caused by different infectious agents. In this case, if the patient has antibodies to EBNA, with or without antibodies to EA, EBV is unlikely to be the cause of the current illness.

An additional, often underdiagnosed, cause of infectious mononucleosis is CMV. It is estimated that CMV is responsible for 20% to 50% of all cases of heterophile-negative mononucleosis.[6] As with EBV, CMV is ubiquitous; many children are asymptomatically infected in early childhood. In immunocompetent adolescents and adults, CMV infection may be subclinical, or it can cause symptoms of infectious mononucleosis. CMV causes significant morbidity and mortality in immunocompromised patients such as organ transplant recipients and people with advanced HIV disease.

Serological testing for CMV is best reserved for those adolescents who present with symptoms of mononucleosis and whose initial testing was not suggestive of acute EBV as the causative agent. Serological testing for CMV in an immunocompetent adolescent consists of measuring both CMV IgM and IgG. A positive CMV-IgM test result is typically diagnostic of primary CMV infection, whereas a positive IgG result indicates previous infection. CMV serological testing is complicated somewhat in that IgM may be present during reactivation of the virus. However, in an otherwise healthy adolescent with symptoms of infectious mononucleosis, a positive CMV-IgM result is strongly suggestive that CMV is the etiology of the mononucleosis. The use of viral culture and quantitative nucleic acid–based testing are usually reserved for use in immunocompromised individuals who have or are at risk for severe disease.

Thus, in a previously healthy adolescent with symptoms of infectious mononucleosis, a reasonable first step for diagnosis is heterophile antibody testing. If heterophile antibodies are detected, no additional testing is necessary. If the heterophile test result is negative, specific serological testing for EBV and CMV should be performed. If these tests fail to yield a diagnosis, additional testing, such as for HIV and/or other etiologies, should be guided by the patient's history and clinical status.

HEPATITIS TESTING

Of the >500 000 cases of acute viral hepatitis diagnosed in the United States each year, 32% are caused by hepatitis A virus (HAV), 43% are caused by hepatitis B virus (HBV), 21% are caused by HCV, and 4% are caused by other or unknown types.[7] The clinical features of acute symptomatic viral hepatitis are similar, regardless of the etiology. There are no clinical features that unequivocally distinguish the individual types of hepatitis from each other; however, epidemiologic patterns of transmission may suggest a particular virus. The incubation period occurs just after acquisition of infection to the time of first symptoms and lasts a few weeks to several months, depending on the etiology. The early symptoms of viral hepatitis include malaise, joint pain, myalgia, fatigue, anorexia, and right upper quadrant abdominal tenderness. For some of these viruses, chronic infection can occur. Knowledge of appropriate serological testing is crucial for determining the etiology of the disease, the expected long-term outcome, and possible therapeutic options for patients.

HEPATITIS A

HAV is most commonly acquired via the fecal-oral route and is often associated with eating food that has been handled by infected individuals. From 1987 through 1997, an average of 28 000 cases of acute hepatitis A disease were reported each year in the United States.[8] These rates have declined significantly since the implementation of hepatitis A vaccine in certain US states. More than half of HAV infections occur among children, which led to the recommendation in 2006 for routine immunization against HAV for all children in the United States. Despite recent immunization successes, a large number of adolescents remain susceptible to infection. A significant risk factor in adolescents is international travel. Infection rates among persons who are unvaccinated before travel departure are estimated to range from 4 to 30 cases per 100 000 months of stay in developing countries.[9]

Serological testing for HAV is most useful in patients who present with symptoms of acute viral hepatitis or in cases for which there is an unexplained elevation of liver enzyme levels in a susceptible patient. Diagnosis of infection is typically established by the detection of IgM antibody to the capsid proteins of the virus. Most often, the IgM anti-HAV becomes detectable 5 to 10 days before the onset of symptoms and persists for 4 to 6 months.[10] Anti-HAV IgG, which appears early in the course of infection, remains detectable for life and provides lifelong immunity against the disease.

HEPATITIS B

HBV is transmitted by exposure to infected blood or other body fluids. In adolescents it is often acquired through unprotected sex and/or intravenous drug

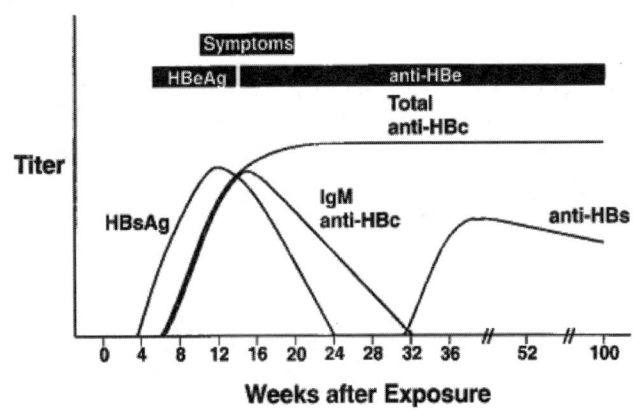

Fig 2. Serological response to HBV infection with recovery. (Reproduced with permission from Long SS. *Principles and Practice of Pediatric Infectious Diseases*. 2nd ed. Philadelphia, PA: Churchill Livingstone, an imprint of Elsevier; 2003: 1090.)

use. A total of 13 829 cases of acute HBV infection were reported in the United States in children and adolescents between 1990 and 2002. The incidence among adolescents aged 15 to 19 years was consistently higher than the incidence in younger children.[11] The clinical presentation is indistinguishable from other causes of viral hepatitis; however, unlike HAV, some individuals develop chronic HBV infection.

Issues such as chronic infection and previous immunization complicate serological testing for HBV. To establish the diagnosis of acute infection, it is necessary to test for hepatitis B surface antigen (HBsAg) and anti-HBV antibodies (Fig 2.). HBsAg is a molecule on the surface of the virus that is detected in serum during acute or chronic hepatitis. The presence of HBsAg indicates that the patient is capable of transmitting infection. HBsAg and IgM antibody to the hepatitis B core antigen (anti-HBc IgM) are usually detectable within 1 to 2 months after infection. Thus, these test results are usually positive as the initial symptoms appear. The presence of anti-HBc IgM is indicative of acute HBV infection, especially when HBsAg is found concurrently. Some patients with HBV also have detectable levels of hepatitis B e antigen (HBeAg). Detectable levels of HBeAg indicate active viral replication with high blood levels of HBV DNA.

As the host antibody response facilitates viral clearance, the HBsAg disappears, indicating the end of acute infection. Disappearance of HBsAg occurs in conjunction with production of anti-HBs antibody. Detectable levels of anti-HBs antibody indicate that the patient has recovered and developed protective immunity to HBV. At approximately the same time, IgG anti-HBc appears and replaces the IgM anti-HBc. When all HBsAg has been neutralized by anti-HBs, there is a brief "window period" where neither HBsAg nor anti-HBs can be detected (Table 1). During this period, the only marker of recent infection is the

Table 1
Serologic pattern for different stages of HBV infection

Stage of Infection	HBsAg	Anti-HBs	IgM anti-HBc	IgG anti-HBc
Incubation period (early)	+	−	−	−
Incubation period (late)	+	−	+	−
Acute hepatitis B	+	−	+	−
Acute hepatitis B (window period)	−	−	+	−
Resolved infection	−	−	−	+
Resolved infection (remote)	−	±	−	+
Chronic infection	+	−	−	+
Hepatitis B vaccination	−	+	−	−
Hepatitis B vaccination (immediately following)	±	−	−	−

+ indicates positive; −, negative. (Reproduced with permission from Long SS. Principles and Practice of Pediatric Infectious Diseases. 2nd ed. Philadelphia, PA: *Churchill Livingstone, an Imprint of Elsevier;* 2003:1090.)

IgM anti-HBc. In persons with resolved HBV infection, IgG anti-HBc remains detectable throughout life, but anti-HBs may become undetectable much later in life. Individuals who have never been infected but have received the HBV vaccine will have anti-HBs but not anti-HBc.

HBV can cause chronic infection. In this case, the anti-HBs is undetectable and the HBsAg test remains positive. Some patients with chronic HBV have persistently detectable levels of HBeAg. The use of quantitative PCR assays for detection of HBV DNA generally is reserved for assessing the degree of viral burden in patients who have chronic infection with HBV. It is not meant to be used as a means of replacing serological assays for diagnosis of hepatitis B disease. Patients with chronic HBV infection are at significant risk of developing cirrhosis and/or hepatocellular carcinoma and, thus, should be referred to a specialist for additional evaluation and care.

HEPATITIS C

Similar to HBV, HCV is also acquired via exposure to infected blood and body fluids. The risk for acquisition is highest in intravenous drug users and commercial sex workers. Testing for HCV infection is recommended for patients who have ever injected illegal drugs, received clotting factors made before 1987, received blood transfusions or organ transplants before July 1992, children born to HCV-positive women, anyone receiving long-term hemodialysis, and health care workers after they have been stuck with a needle, or had mucosal exposure to HCV-positive fluids.[12] Testing is also suggested for victims of sexual assault. In adolescents, testing should be undertaken for any patient who has symptoms consistent with viral hepatitis. HCV infection can be sexually transmitted and, therefore, is a concern for any sexually active teenager. However, routine screening of healthy patients for HCV is not currently recommended.

There is no available IgM antibody test for HCV. The anti-HCV IgG antibody typically becomes detectable 3 to 4 months after infection. The sensitivity and specificity of this test are 97% and 99%, respectively.[13] The IgG antibody test cannot determine if the infection is acute, resolved, or chronic. A positive anti-HCV antibody test must be confirmed with supplemental testing because of the high risk of false-positive test results found when the assay is applied to populations at low risk with no evidence of liver disease. Positive antibody test results are typically confirmed by using the HCV recombinant immunoblot assay (RIBA).[14] The RIBA results are reported as positive, negative, or indeterminate. Alternatively, nucleic acid–based testing can be used to substantiate IgG testing or when HCV-RIBA testing gives indeterminate results. The most commonly used assay is a real-time PCR (RT-PCR). This assay can be used to obtain both qualitative and quantitative measure of HCV viral RNA in serum. When used to confirm antibody testing, a qualitative positive or negative test result is sufficient. The use of quantitative RT-PCR is for monitoring disease and response to treatment in chronically infected patients.

HCV infection is diagnosed when a patient has a positive test result for anti-HCV IgG antibody confirmed with either a positive HCV-RIBA or positive RT-PCR test result. If a positive IgG antibody result is obtained and the RIBA results are indeterminate, both tests should be repeated after 1 month or an RT-PCR should be performed immediately.[15]

HEPATITIS D AND E

Hepatitis A, B, and C are the most commonly encountered forms of viral hepatitis in adolescents; however, it is worth mentioning hepatitis D and E. Hepatitis D virus (HDV) requires the presence of HBV to cause infection. The modes of transmission are the same as those of HBV. Serological testing for HDV is recommended for any teenager who has chronic HBV infection, because infection with HDV increases the risk of cirrhosis and hepatocellular carcinoma. Hepatitis D can be diagnosed by the presence of anti-HDV IgM antibodies.

Hepatitis E virus (HEV) is transmitted via the fecal-oral route and is responsible for sporadic outbreaks in developing countries. Unfortunately, there are no assays for HEV that have been approved for use by the US Food and Drug Administration. Thus, HEV testing should only be performed for teenagers who have a history of foreign travel, symptoms of viral hepatitis, and negative test results for the more common causes of acute hepatitis. HEV antibody assays are available through research laboratories and the Centers for Disease Control and Prevention (CDC).

SYPHILIS

Since 2000, the rates of syphilis have been increasing in the United States. In 2005, the number of reported cases of primary and secondary syphilis (3.0 cases per 100 000 people) was 11.1% higher than in 2004. In 2005, the rates among adolescents varied with ethnicity; rates varied from 0.5 cases per 100 000 people (for non-Hispanic white adolescents) to 9.7 cases (for non-Hispanic black adolescents).[16] The highest increase in syphilis rates occurred among men who have sex with men; these individuals typically exhibit high-risk sexual behaviors and high rates of HIV coinfection. Nevertheless, the rates of syphilis among women have also increased recently. Therefore, all adolescents who present with a history of high-risk sexual behaviors or with any symptoms of a sexually transmitted infection should be screened for syphilis.

The symptoms of primary syphilis include painless ulcers (chancres) of the skin or mucous membranes; however, these lesions may not be recognized. If untreated, secondary syphilis occurs 1 to 2 months later and causes rash, mucocutaneous lesions, and lymphadenopathy. Fever, malaise, sore throat, headache, and arthralgia can be present as well. The rash typically occurs on the palms of the hands and soles of the feet. Secondary syphilis is followed by a variable-length latent period in which there are no active symptoms. Finally, tertiary syphilis occurs years to decades after infection and results in gumma formation involving the skin, bone, viscera, or cardiac system. Neurosyphilis can occur at any stage of the infection.[17] Serological testing for syphilis is usually initiated with the rapid plasma regain (RPR) screening test. The RPR test is much more common and more readily performed than the similar Venereal Disease Research Laboratory slide test. Results of both of these tests become positive ~4 weeks after infection. They are nontreponemal tests: rather than testing for specific anti-*Treponema* antibodies, they test for cross-reactive antibodies to cellular products that are released during infection. Thus, they have a very high false-positive rate. The majority of patients with a false-positive test result will have low RPR titers, with a typical ratio of 1:4 or less. False-negative test results also occur, usually when testing is performed early after infection. Approximately 70% of patients with syphilis will have a positive RPR test result within 2 weeks of the initial symptoms; almost 100% of patients with secondary and latent syphilis will have a positive RPR test result.[17] Thus, any patient with a lesion and/or history that is consistent with syphilis who has a negative RPR test result should have repeat testing performed after several weeks. The rate of RPR test positivity declines during instances of late latent and tertiary disease; however, given the timing involved, this is unlikely to occur during adolescence.[18]

Any patient with a positive RPR or Venereal Disease Research Laboratory test should have specific confirmatory antitreponemal antibody testing (either the fluorescent treponemal antibody absorption test result or the microhemagglutination assay for *Treponema pallidum*). If the antitreponemal antibody test is negative, the RPR test result should be considered false-positive. If the patient has a clinical syndrome consistent with syphilis, treatment should be initiated while awaiting the results of confirmatory testing.

Specific anti-*Treponema* antibody test results are usually positive for life. However, RPR titers can be used to follow the success of treatment and monitor for reinfection. A fourfold decrease in titer within 6 to 12 months of therapy indicates that treatment was successful. If the RPR does not decline, either treatment was not effective or the patient has been reinfected. Typically, RPR testing often becomes negative within 1 year after therapy has been completed. A small proportion of individuals, especially those with high initial titers or those treated later in the course of infection, will have a decrease in titer with therapy but still have persistent positive RPR test results. In either case, a subsequent fourfold rise in titer suggests that reinfection or relapse has occurred. Patients treated for primary, secondary, or early latent syphilis should have follow-up serological testing 6 and 12 months after therapy. Those treated for late latent or tertiary disease should also be tested 24 months after therapy. Any adolescent who exhibits ongoing high-risk sexual behaviors should be tested regularly.

HIV

Infection with HIV continues to be a significant problem in the United States, especially in adolescents. The CDC has estimated that ~40 000 persons become infected with HIV each year, and that many of these infections occur in people between the ages of 13 and 24 years.[19] A recent estimate is that more than half of all HIV-infected adolescents have never been tested for HIV and are unaware of their infection.[20] In 2006, the CDC released new recommendations that suggest that all individuals aged 13 to 64 years who seek any medical care should be tested for HIV. These recommendations are, in part, attributable to the 2004 finding that 39% of patients receiving a diagnosis of AIDS first tested positive for HIV within the preceding 12 months.[20] All patients seeking treatment for sexually transmitted infections should be tested for HIV at each visit regardless of what high-risk behaviors may or may not be present.[20] In addition, all patients starting treatment for *Mycobacterium tuberculosis* should be tested for HIV infection.

There is no uniform law throughout the United States concerning consent and confidentiality for HIV testing in adolescents. It is important to know and adhere to local guidelines when performing testing. HIV screening should be discussed with all adolescents and is strongly encouraged for those who engage in any sexual activity that includes mucosal exposure to any body fluid. HIV testing should especially be considered for teenagers who present with symptoms suggestive of HIV infection, including persistent malaise and fatigue, generalized lymphadenopathy, hepatosplenomegaly, and recurrent diarrhea. Evidence of opportunistic infections with *Candida*, *Pneumocystis*, or other opportunistic infections should always prompt testing.

Initial antibody screening tests for HIV detect IgG antibodies to HIV-1. A negative result rules out HIV infection that occurred up to several months before testing. However, during the early stages of infection, anti-HIV IgG is not yet detectable. This is referred to as the window period during acute infection. During this period, the HIV antibody test result will be negative and the diagnosis can be missed. This period may be as short as 6 weeks with current testing.[21] Nevertheless, it is important to remember that serological testing for HIV may not detect early infection. In cases for which the index of suspicion for early HIV is very high, patients may be screened by using nucleic acid–based testing. Because these tests are not approved for diagnostic testing, they should be ordered and interpreted in conjunction with an infectious disease specialist.

Laboratory samples that test positive for anti-HIV IgG are retested in duplicate. If either of the repeat test results is positive, a confirmatory test must be performed. This confirmatory test is generally a Western blot assay that tests for the presence of anti-HIV IgG with more specificity. If the Western blot result is positive, then the patient is diagnosed with HIV. If the Western blot result is indeterminate, a second test should be performed at least 1 month later. It is often more timely to obtain immediate nucleic acid–based testing. Qualitative PCR testing for HIV RNA can provide a highly sensitive result.

LYME DISEASE

Lyme disease is a bacterial infection caused by *Borrelia burgdorferi*. Infected *Ixodes scapularis* and *Ixodes pacificus* ticks can transmit the bacterium to humans. It is found in certain areas of the United States, including Connecticut, Delaware, Maine, Maryland, Massachusetts, Minnesota, New Hampshire, New Jersey, New York, Pennsylvania, Rhode Island, and Wisconsin. These 12 states account for 95% of the cases reported nationally.[22] Initial Lyme disease testing detects IgM and IgG antibodies against *B burgdorferi*. A positive or equivocal test result must be confirmed by using a Western blot assay. Testing is recommended for patients who live in or have traveled to an endemic area who present with symptoms suggestive of true infection. Clinical infection is divided into 3 phases: early localized disease, early disseminated disease, and late disseminated disease. Early localized disease occurs within the first month after infection and manifests with erythema migrans rash, fever, myalgia, headache, fatigue, regional lymphadenopathy, and arthralgia. Early disseminated disease may present with symptoms similar to early localized disease but may also include multiple areas of erythema migrans rash, generalized lymphadenopathy, conjunctivitis, facial palsy, meningitis, or heart block. Late disseminated disease almost always presents with arthritis. The knee joint is the most commonly involved area of arthritis. Patients with either early or late disseminated disease almost always have a strong IgG response when tested.

Serological testing for Lyme disease should include the use of both IgM and IgG antibody tests. If a patient with a history of residence in or travel to an endemic area has strong clinical evidence of early localized disease and negative initial serology results, the serological tests should be repeated by using acute and convalescent samples to determine if seroconversion has occurred.[23] Normally, IgM antibody to Lyme disease is detectable 3 to 4 weeks after infection and peaks at 6 to 8 weeks. Although IgM levels normally fall after infection, it is not unusual to detect IgM levels for ≥8 months after infection. IgG levels typically peak 3 to 6 months after infection and may provide positive test results indefinitely.[24]

Treatment for Lyme disease may or may not affect antibody levels; therefore, serological testing for Lyme disease cannot be used to evaluate efficacy of therapy or the possibility of infection relapse. However, antimicrobial treatment for Lyme disease is highly effective, and outcomes of patients who receive conventional antibiotic therapy are excellent. Therefore, the most common reason for the "failure" of antibiotic therapy is actually misdiagnosis of a patient who does not have Lyme disease.[24] The difficulty in accurately diagnosing Lyme disease lies in pretest patient selection and interpretation of the Western blot confirmatory assay. Performing Lyme serology in patients with nonspecific symptoms that are not suggestive of Lyme disease, especially in the absence of exposure to an area of high prevalence, significantly increases the chances of a false-positive test result. There are >70 different Food and Drug Administration–approved kits for Lyme disease Western blot testing, and many have different interpretive criteria. The CDC recommends that if the Western blot test is performed, an IgM immunoblot result is considered positive if 2 or more of the following 3 bands are present: 24 kilodaltons (kd) (OspC), 39 kd (BmpA), and 41 kd (Fla). The IgG test result is positive if 5 or more of the following 10 bands are present: 18 kd, 21 kd (OspC), 28 kd, 30 kd, 39 kd (BmpA), 41 kd (Fla), 45 kd, 58 kd (not GroEL), 66 kd, and 93 kd. If the IgM test result is positive but the IgG test result is negative, and the patient has had symptoms for 4 weeks or more before testing, the result is considered false-positive regardless of the bands that are present.

CONCLUSIONS

Serological diagnosis in adolescents is important to understand, because new behaviors and exposures may prompt new patterns of infections in teenagers. As always, obtaining a thorough history and physical examination is imperative. In patients whose symptoms suggest an infectious syndrome, knowledge of appropriate testing is essential. Evaluation of the patient's serum for antibody responses to infectious agents can be a very useful means of diagnosis. The serological principles involved in these tests rely on the host antibody response to the pathogen. Evaluation of an antibody response is frequently sufficient to provide a meaningful diagnosis in the appropriate patient. The nature of the infecting agent and the response of the host can often complicate these tests, and their correct interpretation is crucial. Knowing when to use the appropriate testing in certain clinical circumstances is always the best way to diagnose the diseases accurately.

REFERENCES

1. Ellen Rimsza M, Kirk GM. Common medical problems of the college student. *Pediatr Clin North Am.* 2005;52(1):9-24, vii
2. National Center for Infectious Diseases: Epstein-Barr Virus and Infectious Mononucleosis. Available at: www.cdc.gov/ncidod/diseases/ebv.htm. Accessed March 4, 2008
3. Peter J, Ray CG. Infectious mononucleosis. *Pediatr Rev.* 1998;19(8):276-279
4. Linderholm M, Boman J, Juto P, Linde A. Comparative evaluation of nine kits for rapid diagnosis of infectious mononucleosis and Epstein-Barr virus-specific serology. *J Clin Microbiol.* 1994;32(1): 259-261
5. Hickey SM, Strasburger VC. What every pediatrician should know about infectious mononucleosis in adolescents. *Pediatr Clin North Am.* 1997;44(6):1541-1556
6. Klemola E, Von Essen R, Henle G, Henle W. Infectious-mononucleosis-like disease with negative heterophil agglutination test: clinical features in relation to Epstein-Barr virus and cytomegalovirus antibodies. *J Infect Dis.* 1970;121(6):608-614
7. Curry MP, Chopra S. Acute viral hepatitis. In: Mandell GL, Bennett JE, and Dolin R, eds. *Mandell, Bennett, & Dolin: Principles and Practice of Infectious Diseases.* Vol 1. Philadelphia, PA: Elsevier; 2005:1426-1441
8. Wasley A, Miller JT, Finelli L; Centers for Disease Control and Prevention. Surveillance for acute viral hepatitis: United States, 2005. *MMWR Surveill Summ.* 2007;56(3):1-24
9. Mutsch M, Spicher VM, Gut C, Steffen R. Hepatitis A virus infections in travelers, 1988-2004. *Clin Infect Dis.* 2006;42(4):490-497
10. Bower WA, Nainan OV, Han X, Margolis HS. Duration of viremia in hepatitis A virus infection. *J Infect Dis.* 2000;182(1):12-17
11. Centers for Disease Control and Prevention. Acute hepatitis B among children and adolescents: United States, 1990-2002. *MMWR Morb Mortal Wkly Rep.* 2004;53(43):1015-1018
12. Viral Hepatitis C. Available at: www.cdc.gov/ncidod/diseases/hepatitis/c/plan/Prev_Control.htm. Accessed March 4, 2008
13. American Academy of Pediatrics. Hepatitis C. In: Pickering LK, Baker CJ, Long SS, McMillan JA, eds. *Red Book: 2006 Report of the Committee on Infectious Diseases.* 27th ed. Elk Grove Village, IL: American Academy of Pediatrics; 2006:355-359
14. Fabrizi F, Martin P, Dixit V, et al. Automated RIBA HCV strip immunoblot assay: a novel tool for the diagnosis of hepatitis C virus infection in hemodialysis patients. *Am J Nephrol.* 2001; 21(2):104-111
15. Alter MJ, Kuhnert WL, Finelli L. Guidelines for laboratory testing and result reporting of antibody to hepatitis C virus: Centers for Disease Control and Prevention. *MMWR Recomm Rep.* 2003;52(RR-3):1-13, 15, quiz CE11-CE14
16. Centers for Disease Control and Prevention. Surveillance 2006: national profile (syphilis). Available at: www.cdc.gov/std/stats/syphilis.htm. Accessed March 4, 2008
17. Rawstron S. *Treponema pallidum* (Syphilis). In: Long S, ed. *Principles and Practice of Pediatric Infectious Diseases.* 2nd ed. Philadelphia, PA: Elsevier;2003:954-961
18. Tramont EC. *Treponema pallidum* (Syphilis). In: Mandell GL, Bennett JE, and Dolin R, eds. *Mandell, Douglas, and Bennett's: Principles and Practice of Infectious Disease.* Vol 2. Philadelphia, PA: Elsevier; 2005:2768-2785
19. Centers for Disease Control and Prevention. Basic statistics. Available at: www.cdc.gov/hiv/topics/surveillance/basic.htm. Accessed March 4, 2008

20. Branson BM, Handsfield HH, Lampe MA, et al. Revised recommendations for HIV testing of adults, adolescents, and pregnant women in health-care settings. *MMWR Recomm Rep*. 2006; 55(RR-14):1–17, quiz CE11–CE14
21. Maldarelli F. Diagnosis of human immunodeficiency virus infection. In: Mandell GL, Bennett JE, and Dolin R, eds. *Mandell, Douglas, and Bennett's: Principles and Practice of Infectious Disease*. Vol 1. 6th ed. Philadelphia, PA: Elsevier; 2005:1506–1527
22. Centers for Disease Control and Prevention. Lyme disease: United States, 2001–2002. *MMWR Morb Mortal Wkly Rep*. 2004;53(17):365–369
23. Centers for Disease Control and Prevention. Recommendations for test performance and interpretation from the Second National Conference on serologic diagnosis of Lyme disease. *MMWR Morb Mortal Wkly Rep*. 1995;44(31):590–591
24. Shapiro ED. *Borrelia burgdorferi* (Lyme disease). In: Long S, ed. *Principles and Practice of Pediatric Infectious Diseases*. 2nd ed. Philadelphia, PA: Elsevier; 2003:965–969

Pulmonary Function Testing in the Adolescent

Carol J. Blaisdell, MD*

Department of Pediatrics and Physiology, University of Maryland School of Medicine, W. Lombard Street, Baltimore, MD 21201, USA

Pulmonary function testing can be used as an objective measure of lung function in adolescents and young adults with known or suspected lung disease. Symptoms of dyspnea, chest pain, cough, and wheezing have many potential etiologies. The choice of an appropriate objective and reproducible test of lung function can often confirm a working diagnosis in the clinician's evaluation. In addition, lung function testing is important for assessing progression of lung disease and response to therapy. Some tests are readily available in the primary care office; others should be conducted in a pulmonary function laboratory that follows procedures that have been standardized by the American Thoracic Society[1] and referenced to healthy populations. Indications for pulmonary function testing are listed in Table 1.

PEAK EXPIRATORY FLOW RATE

The peak expiratory flow rate (PEFR) is the most useful measure of lung function in the primary care management of obstructive lung diseases, particularly asthma, because it is inexpensive and can be used at the patient's home or workplace, the clinician's office, and in the acute care setting of the emergency department and hospital. To use a peak flow meter, the adolescent should blow out as quickly as possibly from maximal inhalation (to total lung capacity [TLC]) with his or her mouth closed tightly on the mouthpiece. The highest of 3 attempts should be recorded. It is important to recognize that PEFR performance is effort dependent and a measure of large-airway dysfunction. Patients who do not keep a tight seal on the mouthpiece will produce a falsely low PEFR, and those who put their tongue in the mouthpiece while exhaling (essentially performing a "blow-dart" maneuver) will have falsely elevated PEFR measurements. Consistency of the values with 3 trials at a time suggests reproducible results that can be interpreted.

---

*Corresponding author.
E-mail address: cjblaisdell@comcast.net (C. J. Blaisdell).

Copyright © 2008 American Academy of Pediatrics. All rights reserved. ISSN 1934-4287

Table 1
Indications for spirometry

To determine the nature of the respiratory dysfunction (obstructive vs restrictive disease)
To evaluate respiratory function associated with signs and symptoms
To quantify the extent or progression of known pulmonary disease
To provide an objective measure to determine the appropriateness of reducing therapy for asthma
To measure the effect of occupational exposure
To identify benefits, adverse effects, or consequences of withdrawal of therapy
To assess the presence of airway hyperreactivity
To assess preoperative lung function

Normative data for PEFR for young men and women based on standing height are available to assess flow limitation compared with healthy controls.[2–4] If the values are <80% of the expected or the patient's personal-best PEFR, airflow obstruction should be suspected. This result could be consistent with subjective complaints of an asthmatic patient or may be unexpected in a patient with poor perception of his or her disease.

In a poorly controlled asthmatic patient who frequently accesses acute care in an emergency department, the PEFR can be used to set criteria for contacting the clinician for impending asthma exacerbations. The asthma action plan, which defines adjustment in home asthma management in response to early symptoms of asthma (cough, dyspnea, chest pain), should also have documented the target PEFR for each individual with asthma.[5] The convention is to determine the patient's personal-best PEFR when asthma is under best control in the clinician's office or with home monitoring and to review these data with the provider.

A determination of whether there is significant airflow obstruction for adolescents who complain of exercise-induced dyspnea by using a peak expiratory flow meter can be useful. PEFR monitoring should be reproducible with a minimum of 3 efforts. If there is >20% variability with 3 efforts performed at 1 time, the clinician should suspect that there is a problem with the patient's technique. However, a change of 20% in the PEFR between before and after exercise that elicits dyspnea would be consistent with exercise-induced asthma. PEFR values of >80% of the personal best or expected for height suggest reasonable control if symptoms are absent. When PEFR decreases to <80% of personal best or there is >20% variability from morning to evening PEFR measurements on the same day, then an adjustment of asthma medications would be recommended. Adjustments that could be made include initiating short-acting β-agonist therapy such as albuterol, adding a long-acting β agonist such as salmeterol or formoterol, and/or increasing the dose of inhaled corticosteroid. If PEFR measurements decrease to <50% of the patient's personal best, that would suggest an emergency, and acute care management in an urgent care setting would be appropriate if a dose of short-acting β agonist does not resolve the symptoms and increase the

PEFR back to >50% of the personal best. In this setting, a course of systemic steroids will likely be necessary.

Small-airway disease may be significantly abnormal before the PEFR decreases, so additional monitoring with spirometry is recommended, particularly for adolescents with obstructive lung diseases such as asthma and cystic fibrosis.

SPIROMETRY

Spirometry is the measurement of lung volumes and flows and is the most useful test for determining if respiratory symptoms are attributable to underlying obstructive versus restrictive lung disease. Spirometry does not provide a specific diagnosis; rather, it places a patient in a specific physiologic category if the results are abnormal. Normal spirometry results do not exclude lung disease but can provide reassurance that the disease is not significantly limiting lung function at rest. The most common obstructive lung disease in adolescents is asthma, which affects ~10% of the US population.[6] Cystic fibrosis is also an obstructive lung disease that might present to the clinician with recurrent cough, bronchitis, and/or pneumonia. Restrictive lung diseases include chronic lung diseases that decrease effective lung volumes (eg, bronchopulmonary dysplasia, sickle cell disease), chest wall disorders (eg, scoliosis), and neuromuscular disorders (eg, Duchenne muscular dystrophy).

To distinguish between obstructive and restrictive lung disorders by using spirometry, measures of forced vital capacity (FVC), forced expiratory volume in 1 second (FEV_1), and the ratio of these two (FEV_1/FVC) are a useful start. Patterns of spirometry results are listed in Table 2. The vital capacity is the largest volume of air that a person can either inspire or expire from the lungs. The maneuver required to measure FVC involves taking a maximal inhalation and forcefully exhaling with the mouth tightly closed around a mouthpiece with the nose closed with a nose clip until the entire lung volume is exhaled. The volume exhaled in the first second is the FEV_1 (Fig 1) and will be decreased compared with normal if there is obstruction to exhaled airflow (as with asthma and cystic fibrosis). Flows in the midportion of the forced-exhalation maneuver, forced expiratory

Table 2
Patterns of spirometry results

	Obstructive	Restrictive
FVC	Normal or increased	<80% of predicted
FRC	Increased	Normal or reduced
TLC	Increased	Reduced
FEV_1	Decreased	Normal or increased
FEV_1/FVC	Decreased	Normal or increased
FEF_{25-75}	Decreased	Normal

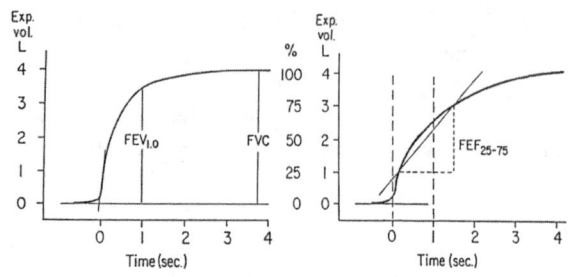

Fig 1. What spirometry measures: FVC (the total volume expired), FEV_1, $FEV_1/FVC\%$ (FEV_1 expressed as a percentage of the FVC), and FEF_{25-75} (the forced midexpiratory flow rate). (Reproduced with permission from Lemen RJ. Pulmonary function testing in the office, clinic, and home. In: Chernick V, Kendig EL, eds. *Kendig's Disorders of the Respiratory Tract in Children*. 5th ed. Philadelphia, PA: WB Saunders; 1990:150.)

flows between 25% and 75% of the FVC (FEF_{25-75}) give an indication of small-airway function and will be the first affected in obstructive lung diseases such as asthma and cystic fibrosis.

The expiratory maneuver that generates the measurements of FEV_1 and FVC is displayed most commonly as a flow-volume loop or can be displayed as a volume-versus-time graph (Fig 2). In obstructive lung diseases, there may be a reduced rate of airflow at any given lung volume. Criteria for assessing for an adequate flow-volume loop include (1) instantaneous start of exhalation and rapid increase in flow to peak, (2) normal sharp peak, indicating maximal effort, (3) smooth, continuous exhalation to zero flow, and (4) reproducible results (Table 3, Fig 3). An unacceptable flow-volume curve is shown in Fig 4, which

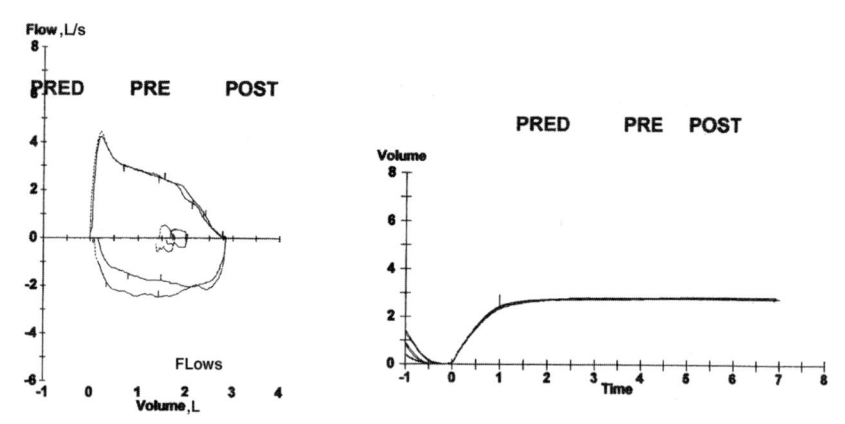

Fig 2. Flow-volume loop and volume versus time of a spirogram. Pulmonary function testing was performed on a Vmax 6200 (SensorMedics, Yorba Linda, CA) at 4 PM. There was good patient effort on the maneuvers. American Thoracic Society criteria were met on spirometry maneuvers, and 2 puffs of albuterol were given via AeroChamber. Pred indicates predicted; Pre, before bronchodilator; Post, after bronchodilator.

Table 3
Characteristics of flow-volume loops

Acceptable flow-volume loop
  Instantaneous start of exhalation and rapid increase in flow to peak
  Normal sharp peak, indicating maximal effort and no large conducting central-airways
    obstruction
  Smooth, continuous exhalation to RV
  Reproducible results
Unacceptable flow-volume loop
  Poor start of exhalation with slow or erratic rise to peak
  Broad or flat peak, which may indicate less-than-optimal effort; if it is smooth and
    reproducible, it may indicate central conducting airway obstructions
  Erratic exhalation with cough or abrupt flow changes
  Exhalation not complete (ie, flow drops abruptly to zero without a gradual return to zero)
  Curve features are not reproducible

demonstrates erratic flows on exhalation attributable to coughing. Without a reliable flow-volume loop, the results of the spirometric maneuver should be in question. The expiratory flow-volume curve provides a more sensitive indication of small-airway obstruction than can be obtained with spirometry. The early reduction of flow and the flattening of the slope are characteristic of obstruction, which appears as a concave expiratory flow tracing (Fig 5). Pulmonary function laboratories should follow standards set by the American Thoracic Society; if they do not, the data should not be trusted.

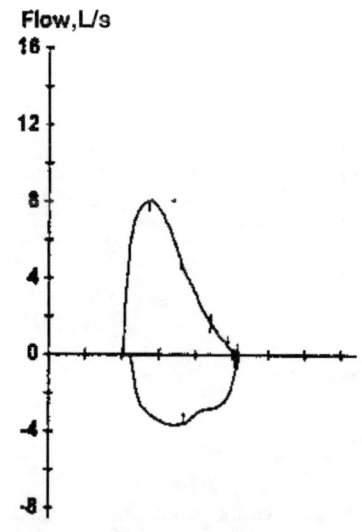

Fig 3. Acceptable flow-volume loop: rapid rise on expiration, a normal sharp peak, smooth exhalation, and gradual return to zero flow.

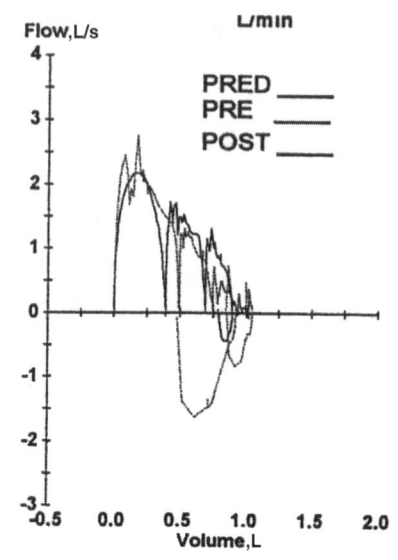

Fig 4. Unacceptable flow-volume loop: poor start, erratic exhalation with cough that lead to inhalation during expiratory phase, and abrupt return to zero. Pred, predicted; Pre, before bronchodilator; Post, after bronchodilator.

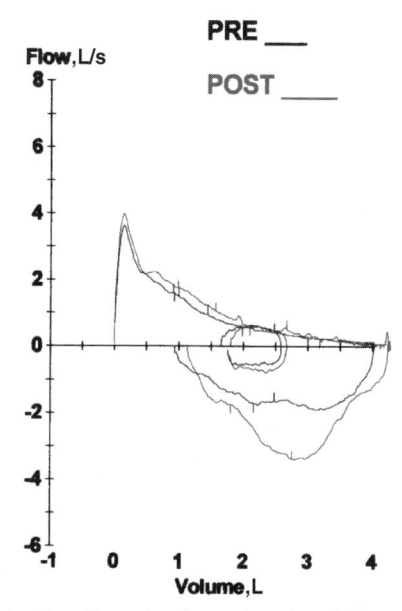

Fig 5. Severe airflow obstruction. Shown is a flow-volume loop demonstrating flow limitation at all lung volumes, with concave tracings on the expiratory loop. Pre indicates before bronchodilator; Post, after bronchodilator. There was no improvement in flows after use of the bronchodilator.

Table 4
Grades of impairment

Grade	FEV$_1$ or FVC, % of That Predicted	FEF$_{25-75}$, % of That Predicted	FEV$_1$/FVC, % of That Predicted
Normal	>80	>70	>75
Mild	<80 to 70	<70 to 60	<75 to 60
Moderate	<70 to 55	<60 to 40	<60 to 40
Severe	<55 to 30	<40 to 15	<40 to 25
Extreme	<30	<15	<25

REFERENCE VALUES

Once the quality of the test is assured, comparisons can be made with reference values from healthy populations, and a determination of the test results can identify patterns of lung function that are consistent with obstructive versus restrictive lung disease. The onset, progression of, or therapeutic correction of lung function abnormalities can also be monitored using objective lung function testing. "Norms" and standards for interpretation[7,8] should be chosen from a study that used a healthy population similar to the population being tested (according to age, gender, and race). If the pulmonary function laboratory does not provide a qualitative interpretation of the data, then fixed-percent predicted cutoffs of <80%, 80%, and 60% are reasonable for identifying abnormalities of FVC, FEV$_1$, and FEF$_{25-75}$, respectively. What is important in the interpretation of lung function testing is knowing that appropriate reference groups were used to determine "abnormal" lung function, because it varies according to age, gender, height, and race. Grades of impairment compared with predicted norms are shown in Table 4. FEV$_1$ or FVC of <80% of that predicted are abnormal. If at 70% to 79%, they are considered mildly abnormal; if at 55% to 69%, they are moderately abnormal; and if they are at 30% to 54%, they are severely abnormal (Table 4). An example of how predicted values can vary depending on the reference group used for comparison is represented in Table 5. For the same spirometry data, using National Health and Nutrition Examination Survey III references[3] for this black teen, FVC and FEV$_1$ were 64% of that predicted, or moderately abnormal. Using the European Respiratory Society (ERS) 1993 standards, which do not include black counterparts, the FVC and FEV$_1$ were 56% and 57% of that predicted, respectively, or moderately severely abnormal.

Women have smaller FEV$_1$ and FVC values at any given age compared with men.[3] In addition, Mexican American and black populations have lower FEV$_1$ and FVC values than do those in the white population at all age groups.[3] The smaller FEV$_1$ values in Mexican American subjects compared with white subjects is related to the shorter standing height of the former for a given age. For

Table 5
Differences of percent-predicted values on spirometry for a black 15-year-old boy

	Subject's Spirometry	Reference (NHANES III, Black)	% Predicted (NHANES III)	Reference ERS 1993	% Predicted ERS 1993
FVC, L	2.69	4.18	64	4.83	56
FEV_1, L	2.29	3.59	64	3.98	57
FEV_1/FVC, % predicted	85	86		83	
FEF_{25-75}, L/s	2.48	4.00	62	5.08	49

NHANES III indicates National Health and Nutrition Examination Survey III; ECRHS, European Community Respiratory Health Survey.

black subjects, the standing height is similar to that of white subjects, but FEV_1 and FVC values are lower in black compared with white and Mexican American subjects.[3] On average, black people have a smaller trunk/leg ratio than do white people, and lung volume depends on chest wall size. This is important to recognize, because lung function values reported on the basis of references that only use white subjects may require a 12% to 15% adjustment factor. This adjustment in the black population if the white references are used is less accurate for determining normal and abnormal ranges of lung function than using appropriate references for the individual on the basis of race, gender, and height. FEV_1 as a percentage of FVC (FEV_1/FVC) is smaller in white compared with Mexican American and black subjects.[3] If a pulmonary function test report suggests a degree of lung function abnormality worse than expected by the clinician, check that the appropriate reference group was used for comparison with the patient's data.

Also important when comparing results in an individual patient over time is to compare absolute volumes and flows and to examine which reference values were used to report the predicted volumes and flows. The use of appropriate references is required not only for spirometry but also for measures of lung volumes and diffusion capacity (see below).

LUNG VOLUMES

When the forced vital capacity on a spirometry test is low (<80% of that predicted), a restrictive lung pattern is suggested if the FEV_1/FVC ratio is normal (>80%) or may reflect air trapping from obstructive lung disease if the FEV_1/FVC is low (<80%). To confirm a restrictive versus obstructive disease pattern, lung volumes that measure the residual volume (RV), functional reserve capacity (FRC), and TLC can be useful (Fig 6). On spirometry, only lung volumes and flow rates within the FVC are measurable: that volume of air that is exhaled or inhaled from maximal inhalation to maximal exhalation, such as the FVC, FEV_1, and FEF_{25-75}. Because RV is the volume of air that cannot be expressed from the

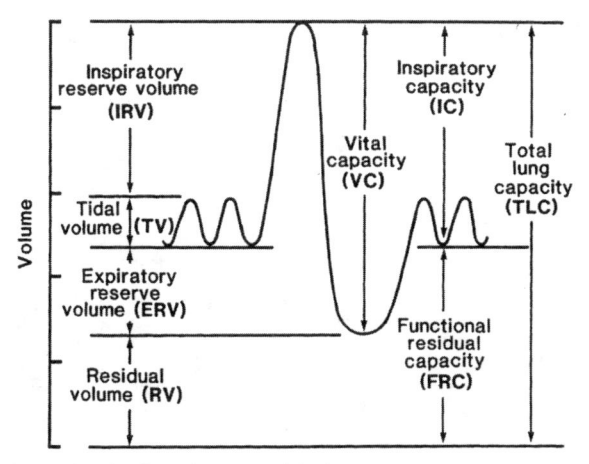

Fig 6. Lung volumes (need to be redrawn as original): RV, amount of air that cannot be expressed from the lung; ERV (expiratory reserve volume), volume that can be exhaled starting from FRC to RV; FRC, the volume of air in the lungs at the end of the tidal breath, and a combination of ERV and RV; TLC, the total volume of air on full inspiration. (Reproduced with permission from Loughlin GM, Eigen H, eds. In: *Respiratory Disease in Children: Diagnosis and Management*. Baltimore: Williams & Wilkins; 1994:79.)

lungs, it must be measured by an indirect method. The most common methods for measuring lung volumes are helium dilution, nitrogen washout, or using body plethysmography (the body box). In practice, the FRC is measured, and RV is back-calculated from the FRC by measurement of the expiratory reserve volume. The helium-dilution and nitrogen-washout methods rely on the mixing of known concentrations of gas with the patient's lung volume at the start of the test, which by convention starts at FRC. If a patient has severe obstructive lung disease, this method is not very accurate, because the gases cannot mix with those regions of the lung that have significant air trapping. In this case, use of the body box is more accurate. Pressure changes at the mouth with the patient inside a closed box determine starting volume (FRC). The body box can provide useful information about air trapping (high FRC or RV) in patients with cystic fibrosis but cannot be used successfully if the patient is too obese to fit in the closed box or is attached to an intravenous pole.

When restrictive lung diseases are suspected, as in neuromuscular disorders and sickle cell disease, requesting lung-volume testing can provide more detail about the severity of the restrictive changes. These studies do take more time than spirometry and must be performed in a pulmonary function laboratory with standardized protocols that follow American Thoracic Society guidelines.

CARBON MONOXIDE DIFFUSING CAPACITY

Carbon monoxide diffusing capacity (DLCO) is the measurement of carbon monoxide (CO) transfer from inspired gas into the pulmonary capillary. The

Age: 15   Height(in): 70   Race: Black   Gender: Male   Weight(lb): 127
Diagnosis: Sickle Cell/ Asthma   Medication:
Dyspnea Rest: No   Dyspnea Exercise: No   Cough: No   Productive (cc):
Persistent: No   Smoker: No   How Long(pk/yrs):   Stopped(yrs):
Cigarettes: No   Cigars: No   Temp: 22   PBar: 757

PULMONARY FUNCTION ANALYSIS

Spirometry

		Ref	Pre Meas	Pre % Ref	Post Meas	Post % Ref	Post % Chg
FVC	Liters	4.83	2.69	56	2.89	60	7
FEV1	Liters	3.98	2.29	57	2.53	64	11
FEV1/FVC	%		83	85		87	
FEF25-75%	L/sec	5.08	2.48	49	3.02	60	22
PEF	L/sec	7.92	5.26	66	5.74	72	9
FET100%	Sec		5.67		6.41		13
FIVC		4.83	2.55	53	2.03	42	-21
FIF50%	L/sec		2.51		1.62		-35
FVL ECode			000011		000000		
MVV	L/min						

Lung Volumes

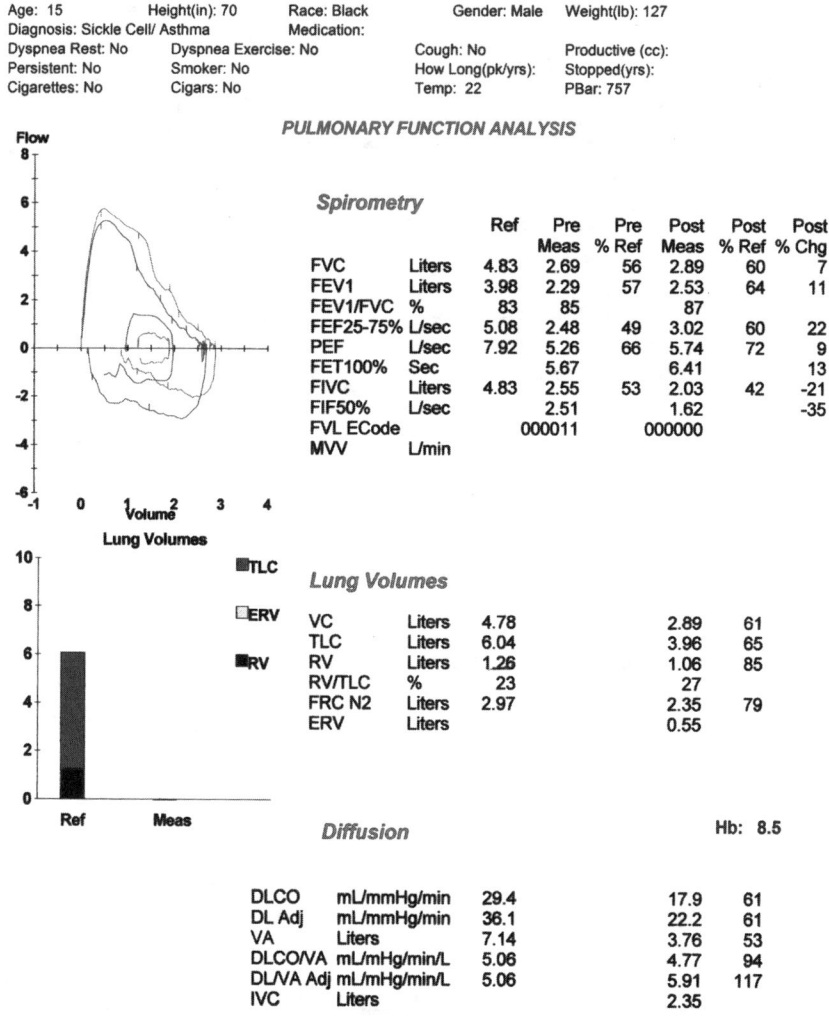

VC	Liters	4.78	2.89	61
TLC	Liters	6.04	3.96	65
RV	Liters	1.26	1.06	85
RV/TLC	%	23	27	
FRC N2	Liters	2.97	2.35	79
ERV	Liters		0.55	

Diffusion

Hb: 8.5

DLCO	mL/mmHg/min	29.4	17.9	61
DL Adj	mL/mmHg/min	36.1	22.2	61
VA	Liters	7.14	3.76	53
DLCO/VA	mL/mmHg/min/L	5.06	4.77	94
DL/VA Adj	mL/mmHg/min/L	5.06	5.91	117
IVC	Liters		2.35	

Fig 7. Example of pulmonary function test: sickle cell disease. Moderate restrictive defect on spirometry is confirmed on lung volumes with FVC of 56% predicted and TLC only 65% of that predicted. Note also that the DLCO is decreased to 61%, corrected for the patient's anemia (with a hemoglobin [Hb] level of 8.5). This patient has had multiple acute chest syndromes.

transfer of CO into the blood depends on the alveolar capillary interface (thickness), capillary volume, hemoglobin concentration, and the reaction rates between CO and hemoglobin.[9] In many diseases, the DLCO correlates with disease severity and arterial blood oxygenation, particularly during exercise.[10] DLCO can be a useful study to examine over time for patients with the potential for progressive loss of alveolar surface area, such as sickle cell disease (see Fig 7), patients with cancer on chemotherapy or radiation therapy, and patients after lung resection. DLCO is diminished in young adults with a history of prematurity regardless of whether they had a diagnosis of bronchopulmonary dysplasia,[11] which likely reflects inadequate growth of the alveoli after premature birth. Normative data for DLCO are not as comprehensively available for ethnic groups and young ages as for spirometry[9]; however, DLCO of 60% to lower limits of normal for the reference population is considered mildly abnormal, 40% to 60% is considered moderately abnormal, and <40% is considered severely abnormal. Trends over time for an individual patient can be evaluated by the clinician to determine if there is progressive loss of alveolar or capillary surface area for gas exchange in certain disease states that need close monitoring, such as patients who are undergoing chemotherapy for cancer and patients with sickle hemoglobinopathy. For example, whole-lung irradiation can lead to mild, moderate, and severe changes in DLCO,[12] so monitoring the effects of therapy for cancer in the adolescent or young adult is very important.

ASSESSING AIRWAY REACTIVITY

Adolescents who have asthma or a history of early neonatal lung injury (eg, bronchopulmonary dysplasia, bronchiolitis, aspiration syndromes, prolonged mechanical ventilation) may have increased bronchial reactivity. In addition, symptoms of dyspnea or chest pain without clear physical findings and normal spirometry at rest, which do not confirm a suspicion of airway obstruction, can be evaluated by using tests of airway reactivity.[13]

Bronchodilator Testing

Spirometry before and after use of a bronchodilator can evaluate the usefulness of bronchodilator therapy for a patient with known or suspected obstructive lung disease (see Fig 8).[14] Asthma is the most common reversible airway obstructive disease, and if it is suspected as the etiology for a patient's signs and symptoms, bronchodilator testing can confirm the diagnosis. For patients with neuromuscular disease, whether bronchodilators would be useful can be assessed with spirometry before and after albuterol use. As shown in Fig 9, a 13-year-old boy with Duchenne muscular dystrophy actually had worse expiratory flows after albuterol use (17% worsening of FEV_1% and 67% worsening of FEF_{25-75}), so albuterol would not be useful in his management. A lack of response to bronchodilator in someone with an obstructive pattern on spirometry should raise questions about a diagnosis of asthma and suggest investigation of alternative disorders such as cystic fibrosis (see Fig 10). Spirometry performed at rest can be repeated 10 to 15 minutes after a standard dose of an inhaled bronchodilator if the patient has not used any bronchodilators for at least 4 hours. Albuterol by metered-dose inhaler (2–4 puffs) with a spacer for adequate dose delivery or 2.5 to 5.0 mg nebulized should be adequate for assessing bronchodilation. An increase in FVC and/or FEV_1 of 12% would be considered a significant bronchodilator response and

A

Age: 15	Height(in): 70	Race: Black	Gender: Male	Weight(lb): 127
Diagnosis: Sickle Cell/ Asthma		Medication:		
Dyspnea Rest: No	Dyspnea Exercise: No		Cough: No	Productive (cc):
Persistent: No	Smoker: No		How Long(pk/yrs):	Stopped(yrs):
Cigarettes: No	Cigars: No		Temp: 22	PBar: 757

PULMONARY FUNCTION ANALYSIS

Spirometry

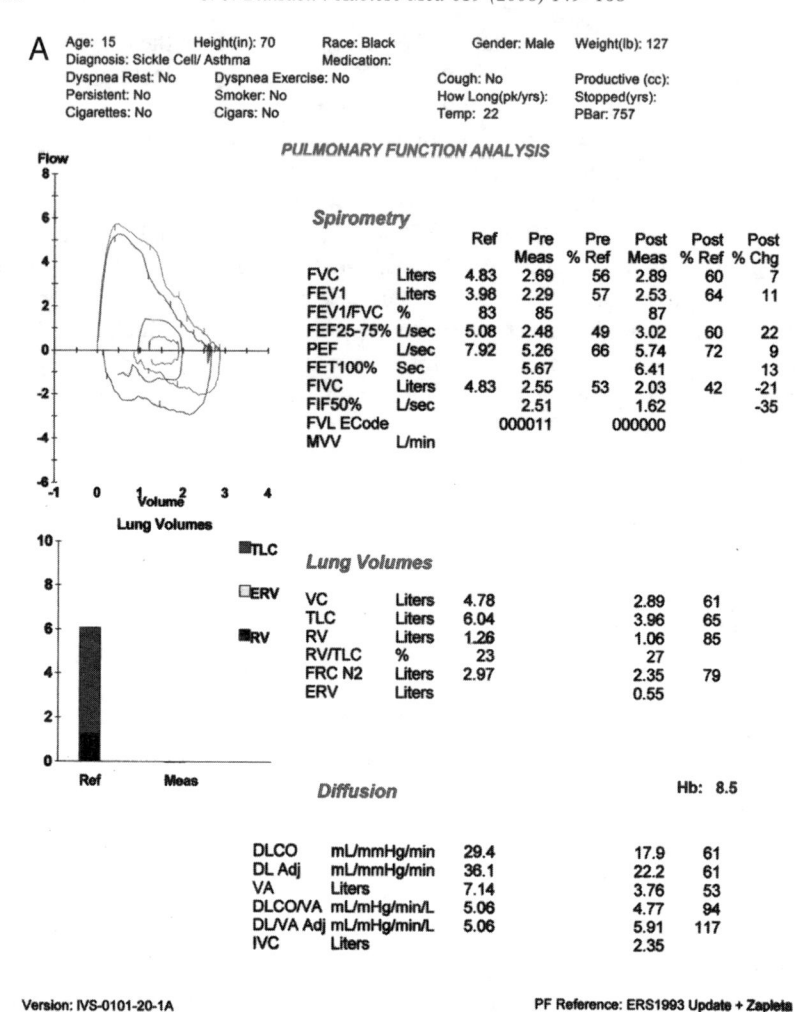

		Ref	Pre Meas	Pre % Ref	Post Meas	Post % Ref	Post % Chg
FVC	Liters	4.83	2.69	56	2.89	60	7
FEV1	Liters	3.98	2.29	57	2.53	64	11
FEV1/FVC	%	83	85		87		
FEF25-75%	L/sec	5.08	2.48	49	3.02	60	22
PEF	L/sec	7.92	5.26	66	5.74	72	9
FET100%	Sec		5.67		6.41		13
FIVC	Liters	4.83	2.55	53	2.03	42	-21
FIF50%	L/sec		2.51		1.62		-35
FVL ECode			000011		000000		
MVV	L/min						

Lung Volumes

		Ref			Meas	% Ref	
VC	Liters	4.78			2.89	61	
TLC	Liters	6.04			3.96	65	
RV	Liters	1.26			1.06	85	
RV/TLC	%	23			27		
FRC N2	Liters	2.97			2.35	79	
ERV	Liters				0.55		

Diffusion

Hb: 8.5

		Ref	Meas	% Ref
DLCO	mL/mmHg/min	29.4	17.9	61
DL Adj	mL/mmHg/min	36.1	22.2	61
VA	Liters	7.14	3.76	53
DLCO/VA	mL/mmHg/min/L	5.06	4.77	94
DL/VA Adj	mL/mmHg/min/L	5.06	5.91	117
IVC	Liters		2.35	

Version: IVS-0101-20-1A   PF Reference: ERS1993 Update + Zapleta

Fig 8. Example of pulmonary function test: severe airflow obstruction attributable to asthma (A) and treated with systemic steroids for 1 week (B). Note improved flows on the second study, and the absence of bronchodilator response on the first study (A) improved on the second study (B) and was best on the third study of the same patient (C), who is a poor perceiver of his asthma.

compatible with a diagnosis of asthma regardless of whether the baseline spirometry test demonstrated obstruction or was normal compared with reference values.

Bronchial Challenge Testing

For those patients with a history or physical examination suggestive of asthma (eg, cough, dyspnea, chest pain, wheezing), it is not uncommon for a clinician to prescribe a trial of bronchodilator and/or an antiinflammatory therapy. However,

B Gender: Male
Age: 15   Race: Black
Height(in): 65   Weight(lb): 128
Diagnosis:

		Ref	Pre	% Ref	Post	% Ref	%Chg
Spirometry							
FVC	Liters	3.44	4.03	117	4.27	124	6
FEV1	Liters	3.00	1.48	49	1.61	54	9
FEV1/FVC	%	86	37		38		
FEF25-75%	L/sec	3.53	0.47	13	0.51	14	8
PEF	L/sec	7.07	3.65	52	4.00	57	10
Vol Extrap	Liters		0.01		-0.01		-222
FVL ECode			000000		001000		

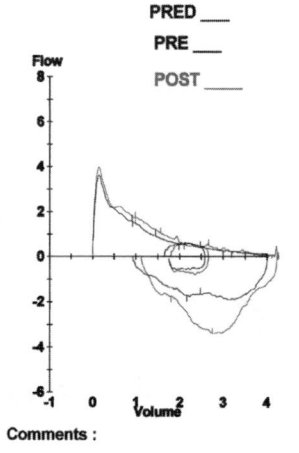

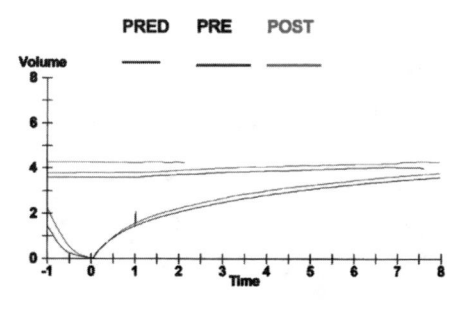

Fig 8. Continued.

continued use of a therapy for an unconfirmed diagnosis of asthma can expose the adolescent to unnecessary adverse effects. When an adolescent with unexplained dyspnea, chest pain, or cough has normal spirometry results and an unclear response to bronchodilators, bronchial challenge testing can be used to diagnose airway hyperreactivity. Airway hyperresponsiveness is likely the most sensitive objective marker of asthma in adolescents and young adults compared with PEFR and spirometry at rest or after bronchodilator use.[15]

Most frequently, inhalation of methacholine is used to determine if airway hyperreactivity compatible with asthma is present. Adolescents with asthma will respond to methacholine with a pattern of airway obstruction on spirometry at a lower dose than nonasthmatic adolescents. In addition to asthma, factors that increase bronchial hyperresponsiveness include exposure to environmental antigens, occupational sensitizers, respiratory infections, air pollutants, cigarette smoke, and chemical irritants.[16] After baseline spirometry is measured, the patient will inhale increasing doses of methacholine. A change in FEV_1 is the primary outcome measure for methacholine challenge testing. The term PC_{20} is

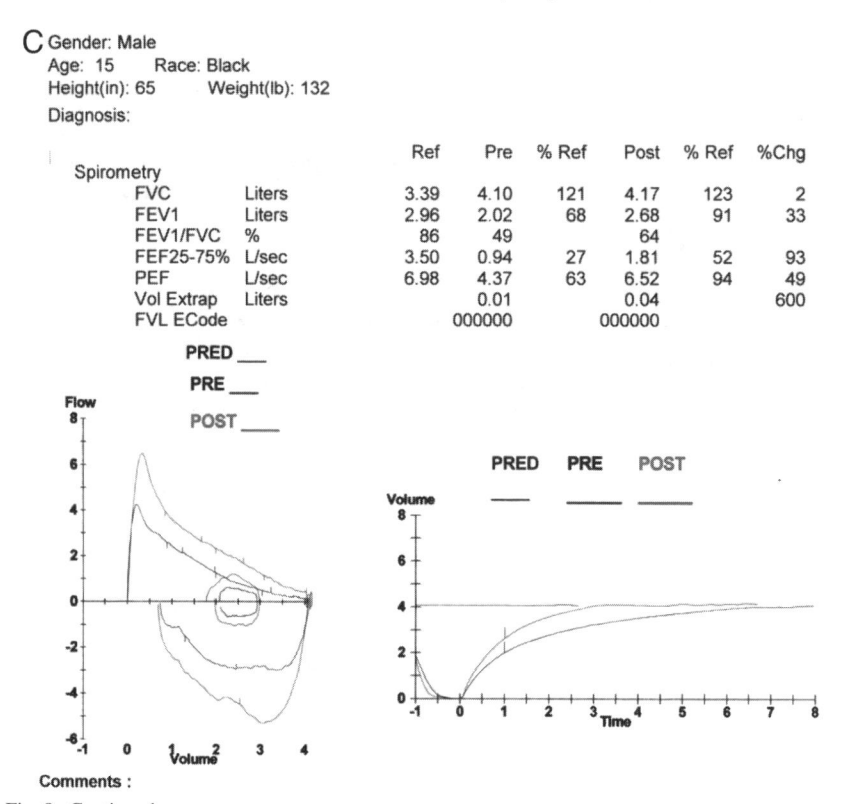

C Gender: Male
Age: 15   Race: Black
Height(in): 65   Weight(lb): 132
Diagnosis:

		Ref	Pre	% Ref	Post	% Ref	%Chg
Spirometry							
FVC	Liters	3.39	4.10	121	4.17	123	2
FEV1	Liters	2.96	2.02	68	2.68	91	33
FEV1/FVC	%	86	49		64		
FEF25-75%	L/sec	3.50	0.94	27	1.81	52	93
PEF	L/sec	6.98	4.37	63	6.52	94	49
Vol Extrap	Liters		0.01		0.04		600
FVL ECode			000000		000000		

Comments :

Fig 8. Continued.

defined as the exact concentration of methacholine that causes a 20% drop in FEV_1 from the baseline FEV_1. A positive test is one in which the PC_{20} is <4.0 mg/mL (Table 6; see ref [16]). If the patient has a PC_{20} of <1.0 mg/mL, he or she has moderate-to-severe bronchial hyperreactivity. If doses of >16 mg/mL methacholine do not cause a 20% drop in FEV_1, then the patient is considered normal, and another etiology for the reported symptoms should be sought. Approximately 30% of patients without asthma who have allergic rhinitis will have a PC_{20} in the borderline range (4.0–16 mg/mL). Approximately 90% to 98% of asthmatic patients will be hyperreactive to methacholine or histamine (another inhalation challenge agent).[17] Methacholine challenge testing should be performed in a pulmonary function laboratory with experienced personnel, because risks of serious airflow obstruction exist.

EXERCISE CHALLENGE TESTING

Although a little less sensitive than methacholine, bronchial challenge testing can also be accomplished by using exercise on a treadmill or bicycle. The test may

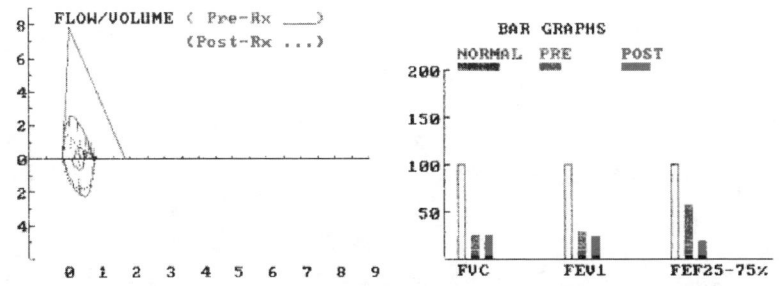

Fig 9. Example of pulmonary function test: Duchenne muscular dystrophy. A severe restrictive pattern is shown, with FVC at only 0.96 L or 26% of that predicted, FEV$_1$ at 0.90 L or 28% of that predicted, and FEV$_1$/FVC at 94%, with worsening after bronchodilator (17% decreased FEV$_1$ [post-Rx]).

be particularly useful for a patient whose respiratory complaints occur primarily with exercise to confirm a suspected diagnosis of exercise-induced asthma or bronchoconstriction (EIB) (used interchangeably), determine the ability of a young adult to perform demanding or life-saving work, and determine the effectiveness of therapy to prevent symptoms. EIB occurs in as many as 95% of asthmatic children and adolescents[18,19] and cannot be excluded on the basis of a negative response to methacholine. An adolescent with suspected EIB who does not respond to pretreatment with a bronchodilator and who has no other manifestations of asthma should be referred for exercise challenge testing to confirm the diagnosis rather than continue to expose the patient to potentially harmful adverse effects.[13]

Patients are asked to walk and/or run on a treadmill to reproduce symptoms experienced with exercise. A minimum of 4 minutes at the target heart rate or ventilation is standard. For the bicycle ergometer to accomplish an adequate test, a target work rate to achieve the target ventilation must be sustained for at least

CYSTIC FIBROSIS

Age: 21 Years
Sex/Race: Female / Caucasian
Height: 59 in 150 cm
Weight: 86 lbs 39 kg

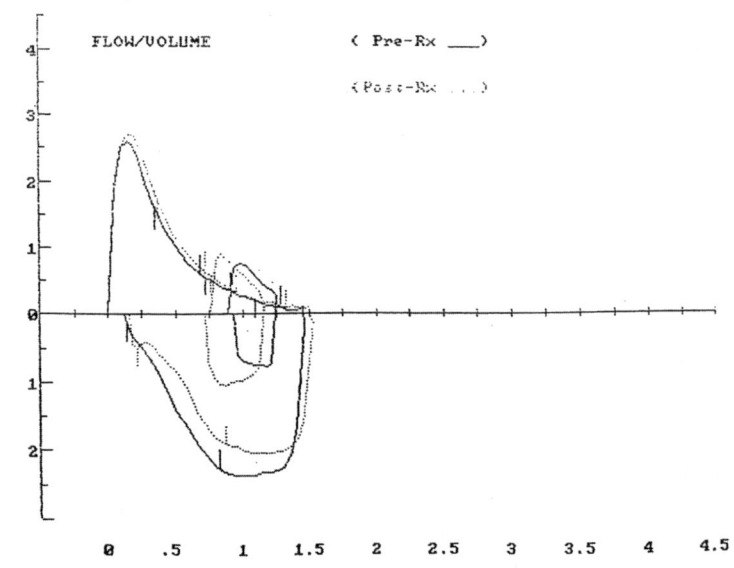

	SPIROMETRY (BTPS)	PRED	PRE-RX BEST	%PRED	POST-RX BEST	%PRED	%CHG
FVC	Liters	3.31	1.45 #	44*	1.52 #	46*	5
FEV1	Liters	3.01	0.91 #	30*	0.94 #	31*	3
FEV1/FVC	%	91	63 #	69*	62 #	68*	-2
FEF25-75%	L/Sec	4.02	0.48 #	12*	0.46 #	11*	-4
FEF25%	L/Sec		1.48		1.63		10
FEF50%	L/Sec		0.54		0.56		4
FEF75%	L/Sec		0.20		0.16		-20
PEF	L/Sec		2.60		2.75		6
FIVC	Liters	3.31	1.33 #	40*	1.37 #	41*	3
PIF	L/Sec		2.38		2.64		11

\# = OUTSIDE 95% CONFIDENCE INTERVAL   * = OUTSIDE NORMAL RANGE
IPS-OL01-05 IPS-OL02-05 N-2103-3

Fig 10. Example of pulmonary function test: cystic fibrosis. Shown are severe airflow obstruction (FEV$_1$ at 30% of that predicted) and a severe restrictive pattern (FVC at 44% of that predicted), with no improvement after bronchodilator administration. Note that flow limitation is worse with forced exhalation compared with tidal breathing at rest.

4 to 6 minutes. As with methacholine challenge testing, the change in FEV$_1$ is the primary outcome variable. Repeated measures of spirometry are performed immediately after exercise and then serially 5, 10, 15, and 20 minutes after completing the exercise. If the FEV$_1$ is not back to a baseline level by 20 minutes, then another measure at 30 minutes should be taken. Response to a bronchodilator may be assessed if the patient experiences significant dyspnea or the FEV$_1$ has not returned to within 10% of baseline at 30 minutes. A 10% decrease from

Table 6
Methacholine challenge interpretation of bronchial hyperresponsiveness

PC_{20}	Interpretation
>16 mg/mL	Normal
4–16 mg/mL	Borderline
1–4 mg/mL	Mild
<1 mg/mL	Moderate to severe

the baseline FEV_1 is generally accepted as abnormal,[19,20] although a decrease of 15% is considered by some to be more diagnostic of EIB.[13,21]

CARDIOPULMONARY EXERCISE TESTING

Cardiopulmonary exercise testing (CPET) involves the assessment of cardiac and pulmonary function during incremental exercise and includes measurements of gas exchange (oxygen consumption, carbon dioxide production, minute ventilation), an electrocardiogram, and blood pressure measurement.[22] The clinician would request such a test for patients who complain of shortness of breath, dyspnea on exertion, or exercise intolerance without a clear etiology or response to therapeutic trials. If the patient has chest pain or symptoms suggestive of cardiovascular disease, a cardiac stress test should be performed by a cardiologist. Exercise challenge testing would be more appropriate if the patient complains of chest tightness and wheezing during or after exercise (see "Exercise Challenge Testing" above). CPET is useful for an adolescent who feels limited by exercise. Limitation can be attributable to impaired lung function, impaired cardiac, pulmonary, or peripheral circulation, or poor conditioning. Patients with asthma, chronic lung disease, or sickle cell disease may have limitations to their oxygenation or ventilatory responses to exercise. CPET should be considered for the following indications: determination of exercise capacity or the cause of any exercise impairment, identification of abnormal responses to exercise, risk stratification and exercise response for training and rehabilitation, evaluation of results of treatment, preoperative assessment, impairment/disability evaluation, and unexplained dyspnea.

PULSE OXIMETRY

Pulse oximetry is a convenient, in vivo, noninvasive technique for measuring oxygen saturation. Oxygen saturation is determined by the ratio of oxyhemoglobin to the sum of oxyhemoglobin and reduced hemoglobin. Pulse oximeters perform optical measurements across a pulsating arterial bed (the finger, ear) at only 2 wavelengths of light to discriminate oxygenated and deoxygenated hemoglobin. Carboxyhemoglobin and methemoglobin also absorb light at the wavelengths measured by the pulse oximeter and, if abundant, can affect the accuracy of the pulse oximeter. These devices were calibrated by using healthy volunteers with insignificant amounts of dysfunctional hemoglobins.[23]

Pulse oximetry is used widely to assess arterial oxygenation and provides a useful estimate of hypoxia. Oxygen saturations of <93% predict a Pao_2 of <70 mm Hg. The pulse oximeter has been validated in various cohorts of patients with presumably normal hemoglobin levels, such as neonates, and in patients with cyanotic heart disease.[24] A retrospective review of simultaneous pulse oximetry and arterial blood gas analysis data obtained from patients with sickle cell disease in the emergency department suggested that the pulse oximeter did not predict hypoxemia well.[25] In addition, a prospective study of children and adolescents with sickle cell hemoglobin demonstrated that pulse oximetry overestimated the number of children with hypoxia[26] and could have led to inappropriate treatment with supplemental oxygen.

Reliance on the pulse oximeter for assessing normoxia in an adolescent or young adult with potential smoke inhalation is inappropriate. Carbon monoxide bound to hemoglobin has similar wavelength-absorption characteristics as oxygenated hemoglobin. Therefore, patients with smoke inhalation will have a falsely normal pulse oximetry value. In the evaluation of a patient with potential smoke exposure, the measurement of carboxyhemoglobin directly from an arterial blood sample is essential. Methemoglobin causes the pulse oximeter readout to tend toward 85%. If the clinician is aware of the presence of dyshemoglobins in the blood of an individual patient, correlation of an arterial blood sample with pulse oximetry would be advisable. It is important to remember that normal oxygen saturation of the blood does not ensure adequate oxygen delivery to the tissues. This is especially true in anemic patients, patients in heart failure, or patients in shock.

ARTERIAL BLOOD GAS

Arterial blood gas (ABG) measurements are used to assess oxygenation and ventilation. Although the pulse oximeter indirectly measures oxygenation by displaying a predicted oxygen saturation, the ABG can provide direct measures of hemoglobin oxygen saturation (measured $HgbO_2sat$), pH, Pao_2, $Paco_2$. These values are extremely important in assessing patients with acute respiratory distress, smoke inhalation, or cyanosis before respiratory failure ensues. The ABG values will guide interventions and monitoring to be performed in the most appropriate setting (office, emergency department, hospital ward, or ICU). Response to therapy can then be reassessed by using the ABG values.

The $Paco_2$ reflects adequacy of ventilation. $Paco_2$ is very tightly regulated under normal circumstances, with values usually between 40 and 42 mm Hg. When a patient is tachypneic, the $Paco_2$ will decrease inversely proportional to the rise in respiratory rate. If an adolescent has a respiratory rate of 12/minute when well and increases his or her respiratory rate during an asthma exacerbation to

24/minute, there would be an expected decline in Pa_{CO_2} measured on an ABG test. If the Pa_{CO_2} in such a setting is 45 mm Hg, the patient has impending respiratory failure and should be transferred to an acute care setting immediately. One should not be reassured that the Pa_{CO_2} is slightly elevated in this situation. This would be just as dangerous as assessing that an adolescent is stable when he or she has absent breath sounds and is no longer wheezing. In acute disease, the pH will decrease in proportion to the rising Pa_{CO_2}. For every 10 mm Hg increase in Pa_{CO_2}, the pH would be expected to drop by 0.04. If the pH is even lower than that expected from the measured Pa_{CO_2}, then metabolic acidosis has also occurred.

In adolescents with chronic lung disease, the Pa_{CO_2} may be elevated and the pH normal. This occurs over days and weeks by alkalinizing the blood with bicarbonate and is metabolic compensation of respiratory acidosis. This would be seen in moderate-to-severe states of cystic fibrosis and neuromuscular disorders as the disease progresses. This would not be expected in young adults with obstructive sleep apnea, who have significant CO_2 retention attributable to upper-airway obstruction, because the hypercarbia should only occur with sleep, and ventilation normalizes when the patient is awake.

REFERENCES

1. Miller MR, Crapo R, Hankinson J, et al. General considerations for lung function testing. *Eur Respir J.* 2005;26(1):153–161
2. Hsu KH, Jenkins DE, Hsi BP, et al. Ventilatory functions of normal children and young adults: Mexican-American, white, and black. I. Spirometry. *J Pediatr.* 1979;95(1):14–23
3. Hankinson JL, Odencrantz JR, Fedan KB. Spirometric reference values from a sample of the general U.S. population. *Am J Respir Crit Care Med.* 1999;159(1):179–187
4. Radeos MS, Camargo CA Jr. Predicted peak expiratory flow: differences across formulae in the literature. *Am J Emerg Med.* 2004;22(7):516–521
5. National Heart, Lung and Blood Institute. New NHLBI guidelines for the diagnosis and management of asthma. *Lippincott Health Promot Lett.* 1997;2(7):1, 8–9
6. Mannino DM, Homa DM, Akinbami LJ, Moorman JE, Gwynn C, Redd SC. Surveillance for asthma: United States, 1980–1999. *MMWR Surveill Summ.* 2002;51(1):1–13
7. Pattishall EN. Pulmonary function testing reference values and interpretations in pediatric training programs. *Pediatrics.* 1990;85(5):768–773
8. Pellegrino R, Viegi G, Brusasco V, et al. Interpretative strategies for lung function tests. *Eur Respir J.* 2005;26(5):948–968
9. Macintyre N, Crapo RO, Viegi G, et al. Standardisation of the single-breath determination of carbon monoxide uptake in the lung. *Eur Respir J.* 2005;26(4):720–735
10. Zapletal A, Houštěk J, Samánek M, Copová M, Paul T. Lung function in children and adolescents with idiopathic interstitial pulmonary fibrosis. *Pediatr Pulmonol.* 1985;1(3):154–166
11. Vrijlandt EJ, Gerritsen J, Boezen HM, Grevink RG, Duiverman EJ. Lung function and exercise capacity in young adults born prematurely. *Am J Respir Crit Care Med.* 2006;173(8):890–896
12. Weiner DJ, Maity A, Carlson CA, Ginsberg JP. Pulmonary function abnormalities in children treated with whole lung irradiation. *Pediatr Blood Cancer.* 2006;46(2):222–227
13. Abu-Hasan M, Tannous B, Weinberger M. Exercise-induced dyspnea in children and adolescents: if not asthma then what? *Ann Allergy Asthma Immunol.* 2005;94(3):366–371
14. Miller MR, Hankinson J, Brusasco V, et al. Standardisation of spirometry. *Eur Respir J.* 2005;26(2):319–338

15. Ulrik CS, Postma DS, Backer V. Recognition of asthma in adolescents and young adults: which objective measure is best? *J Asthma.* 2005;42(7):549–554
16. Crapo RO, Casaburi R, Coates AL, et al. Guidelines for methacholine and exercise challenge testing: 1999. This official statement of the American Thoracic Society was adopted by the ATS Board of Directors, July 1999. *Am J Respir Crit Care Med.* 2000;161(1):309–329
17. Chai H, Farr RS, Froehlich LA, et al. Standardization of bronchial inhalation challenge procedures. *J Allergy Clin Immunol.* 1975;56(4):323–327
18. Godfrey S. Exercise-induced asthma: clinical, physiological, and therapeutic implications. *J Allergy Clin Immunol.* 1975;56(1):1–17
19. Backer V, Ulrik CS. Bronchial responsiveness to exercise in a random sample of 494 children and adolescents from Copenhagen. *Clin Exp Allergy.* 1992;22(8):741–747
20. Cropp GJ. Relative sensitivity of different pulmonary function tests in the evaluation of exercise-induced asthma. *Pediatrics.* 1975;56(5 pt 2):860–867
21. Haby MM, Anderson SD, Peat JK, Mellis CM, Toelle BG, Woolcock AJ. An exercise challenge protocol for epidemiological studies of asthma in children: comparison with histamine challenge. *Eur Respir J.* 1994;7(1):43–49
22. American Thoracic Society; American College of Chest Physicians. ATS/ACCP statement on cardiopulmonary exercise testing [published correction appears in *Am J Respir Crit Care Med.* 2003:1451–1452]. *Am J Respir Crit Care Med.* 2003;167(2):211–277
23. Yelderman M, New W Jr. Evaluation of pulse oximetry. *Anesthesiology.* 1983;59(4):349–352
24. Poets CF, Southall DP. Noninvasive monitoring of oxygenation in infants and children: practical considerations and areas of concern. *Pediatrics.* 1994;93(5):737–746
25. Goepp J, Murray C, Walker A, Simone E. Oxygen saturation by pulse oximetry in patients with sickle cell disease: lack of correlation with arterial blood gas measurements [abstract]. *Pediatr Emerg Care.* 1991;7:387
26. Blaisdell CJ, Goodman S, Clark K, Casella JF, Loughlin GM. Pulse oximetry is a poor predictor of hypoxemia in stable children with sickle cell disease. *Arch Pediatr Adolesc Med.* 2000;154(9):900–903

Cardiac Testing in Adolescents

Christian D. Nagy, MD, W. Reid Thompson, MD*

Division of Pediatric Cardiology, Department of Pediatrics, The Helen B. Toussig Congenital Heart Disease Center, Johns Hopkins University School of Medicine, Brady 5th Floor, 600 N. Wolfe Street, Baltimore, MD 21287, USA

Diagnostic testing in adolescents and young adults with known or suspected heart disease typically involves the use of electrocardiography, various imaging modalities, and, in some cases, other laboratory investigations. In this article we discuss common tests that may be ordered by the generalist or cardiologist to evaluate the heart. The emphasis is on indications for ordering a specific test, understanding the strengths and weaknesses of those tests, and basic interpretation of the results. Heart disease in adolescents primarily includes previously diagnosed congenital lesions, undiagnosed defects (such as atrial septal defect or aortic valve abnormalities) that are often asymptomatic in childhood, inherited latent conditions that may first become manifest during the teenage years (such as hypertrophic cardiomyopathy [HCM]), and acquired disease such as myocarditis. Signs and symptoms of possible heart disease, when present, may include a pathologic murmur or heart sound(s), chest pain and shortness of breath, especially when associated with exercise, palpitations or syncope, or signs of heart failure such as a gallop, increased jugular venous distension, hepatomegaly, rales, and peripheral edema. Often, a careful family history may yield important clues to the possibility of inherited cardiac disease. An electrocardiogram (ECG) is often ordered by the generalist or specialist to evaluate symptoms of possible heart disease or to monitor potential adverse effects of medications. Most imaging studies, including echocardiography, cardiac MRI, computed tomography (CT), and cardiac catheterizations are ordered or performed by the cardiologist to diagnose specific defects or conditions, and catheterizations increasingly are performed primarily for intervention purposes.

ELECTROCARDIOGRAPHY

The ECG remains an invaluable noninvasive tool for assessing the electrical activity of the heart to evaluate adolescents with known or suspected cardiovas-

---

*Corresponding author.
E-mail address: wthomps2@jhmi.edu (W. R. Thompson).

cular disease and may be appropriately ordered by the generalist as part of the investigation of symptoms or monitoring of therapy. The standard 12-lead ECG helps to identify abnormalities of impulse formation (sinus bradycardia, isolated premature atrial, junctional, or ventricular beats, or atrial, junctional, or ventricular arrhythmias) or impulse propagation such as slowed conduction through the atrioventricular (AV) node (AV block) and His-Purkinje system (high-degree AV block or bundle-branch blocks). It can identify those individuals with a short PR interval and delta wave, which indicates ventricular preexcitation (Wolff-Parkinson-White syndrome [WPW]). Repolarization syndromes that involve abnormal myocardial cell membrane ion channels (long QT syndrome [LQTS] and Brugada syndrome) can also be diagnosed on the standard ECG. In addition, abnormalities of the ECG associated with hypertrophic cardiomyopathy, inflammation (myocarditis or pericarditis), myocardial ischemia (anomalous coronary arteries or premature coronary artery disease), or injury (myocardial infarction) can be detected. Serial ECGs are also commonly used to monitor potential cardiac effects of certain psychotropic medications.

Guidelines for the performance of ECGs were published by the American College of Cardiology and American Heart Association (ACC/AHA) in 1992[1] and have not changed in recent years. These guidelines make recommendations for the use of ECGs in patients with and without cardiovascular disease, which for the most part, are applicable to the adolescent population.[2]

Electrocardiography is a quick, inexpensive, and widely available test that can be administered accurately in a variety of clinical settings with a minimum of training. In addition, detailed automated computer interpretation algorithms can assist in interpretation, although the results must always be carefully confirmed for accuracy by an experienced reader. Data can be stored digitally and transmitted electronically or by fax for rapid expert interpretation. Artifacts include those attributable to movement or faulty connections, although many errors in connection can be detected easily (eg, by checking for consistency between lead I versus V6 pattern). The ECG is less helpful for diagnosing specific structural abnormalities and has a high false-positive rate for detecting left-ventricular hypertrophy, particularly in athletes or those with thin body habitus.

Interpretation of Abnormal Heart Rate and Rhythm

Sinus tachycardia, which is characterized by a heart rate that is >98th percentile for age (usually more than 120 but less than ~200 beats per minute with P waves of normal axis [0°–90°]) preceding each QRS complex, is by far the most common tachyarrhythmia and is often attributable to an underlying hypersympathetic state such as fever, pain, anxiety, anemia, dehydration, substance abuse or withdrawal, or hyperthyroidism. Other forms of narrow complex tachycardia represent primary cardiac disorders of either increased

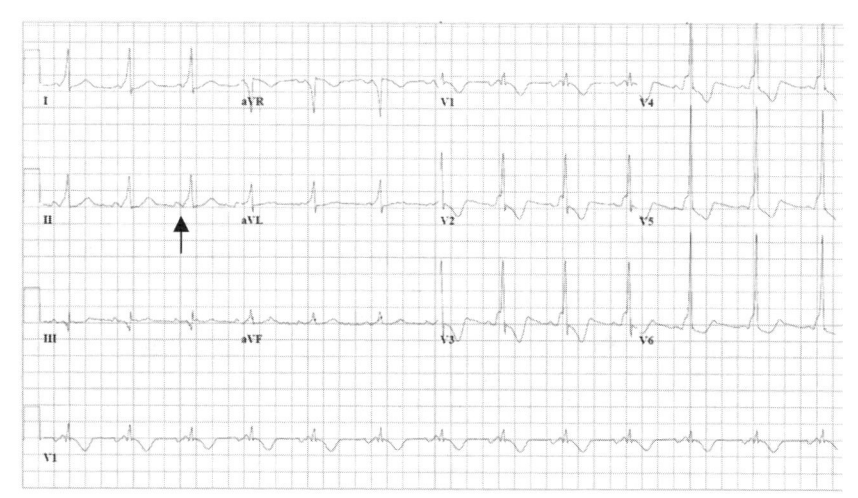

Fig 2. ECG of a 20-year-old woman with WPW. Note the short PR interval and the upstroke (delta wave) from the end of the P wave to the beginning of the QRS complex (arrow).

automaticity or reentry pathways. When the atrial activity (P wave) occurs shortly after the QRS complex, an atrioventricular bypass tract is the most likely mechanism (Fig 1). The baseline (nontachycardic) ECG in patients with WPW shows the typical short PR interval with an upstroke (delta wave) from the end of the P wave to the beginning of the QRS (Fig 2). When a regular, narrow complex tachycardia is present with no visible P waves, simultaneous depolarization of the atria and ventricles with the P wave "hidden" in the QRS complex is more likely, which indicates an AV nodal reentry tachycardia. When P waves are present before the QRS but have an

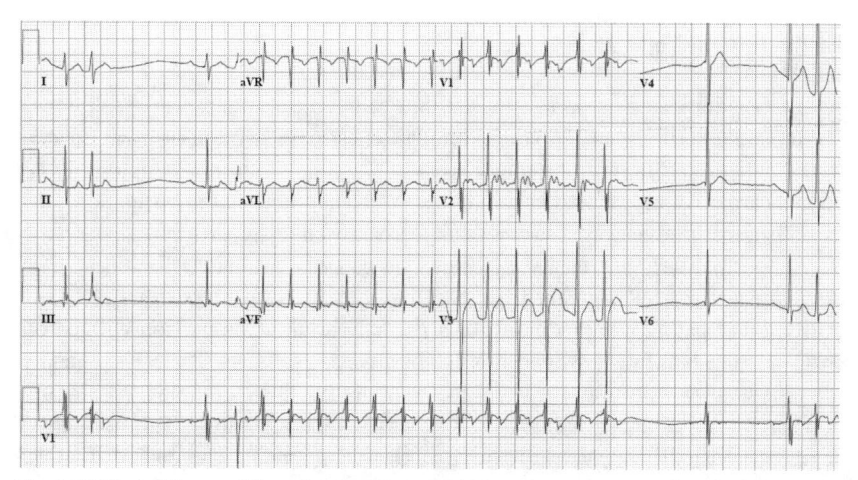

Fig 1. ECG of a 13-year-old boy showing supraventricular tachycardia alternating with bradycardia.

abnormal axis (ie, other than 0°–90°), automatic or ectopic atrial tachycardias are more likely. When the 12-lead ECG demonstrates a wide complex tachycardia (QRS duration of >120 milliseconds), the differential diagnosis includes ventricular tachycardia (VT), supraventricular tachycardia with aberrant conduction between the atria and ventricles, or a fixed bundle-branch block.

Bradycardia in the adolescent is seen in competitive athletes and individuals with eating disorders (eg, anorexia nervosa) and is most commonly manifested on an ECG as sinus bradycardia (defined as sinus rhythm with a heart rate of <2nd percentile for age, usually at <60 beats per minute). Other causes of sinus bradycardia include hypoxia, hypothyroidism, hypothermia, hypercalcemia, hyperkalemia, hypoglycemia, and increased intracranial pressure. In addition, bradycardia may be seen in congenital LQTS. In patients with complete heart block (CHB), the ventricular rate is slower and dissociated from the atrial rate (Fig 3). CHB occurs congenitally in infants born to mothers with lupus or may be acquired after certain infections (eg, Lyme disease).

Adolescents being evaluated for palpitations or syncope should have an ECG performed as a simple, inexpensive, and noninvasive diagnostic tool. Ideally, a 12-lead ECG should be recorded during an episode of symptoms, although this is often not feasible. Approximately up to 50% of patients evaluated for syncope will have an abnormal but nondiagnostic ECG result.[3] The presence of ventricular preexcitation, ectopic atrial or ventricular beats, ventricular hypertrophy, long QT interval, bradycardia, or sustained tachycardia suggests a plausible cause of syncope. Premature ventricular beats (Fig 4) are common findings and usually do not require additional investigation. If they occur with increased frequency, a Holter monitor can aid in quantification, and an echocardiogram is useful for excluding ventricular dysfunction.

Evaluation of Chest Pain

An ECG is indicated as part of the initial evaluation of adolescents with nonreproducible, exertional chest pain. Although chest pain is often of great concern to the patient and family, the majority of adolescents with this symptom do not have a cardiac etiology. ECG changes that warrant additional investigation, such as ST-segment deviation, T-wave changes, ventricular hypertrophy, or conduction abnormalities, are easily detected. In patients evaluated for chest pain, deviations of the ST segment from baseline may indicate myocardial ischemia, injury, other pathologic processes, or a normal variant. Comparison with an old ECG is often helpful; however, this is not always available. The ST segment is identified as the portion between the end of the QRS complex (ventricular depolarization) and beginning of the T wave (repolarization). The normal ST segment is usually isoelectric relative to the TP segment. The end of the QRS complex is marked by the junction to the ST segment (J point) (Fig 5).

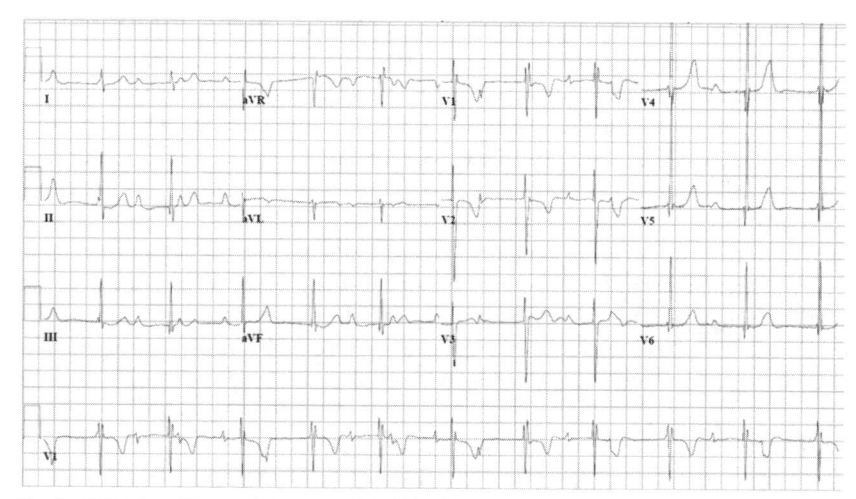

Fig 3. ECG of an 18-year-old woman with CHB. The P waves regularly march out at a higher rate than the QRS complexes.

Variations occur in the ST pattern. It is important to recognize them, because they can be mistaken for abnormalities. ST-T patterns can be affected by changes in autonomic tone, variations in body position, hyperventilation, drinking cold water, and performing Valsalva maneuvers. ST-segment elevation in adolescents may represent benign early repolarization or be seen with pericarditis, acute myocardial infarction (eg, in the setting of cocaine use), commotio cordis, left-ventricular hypertrophy, left bundle-branch block, hyperkalemia, and critical illness (including neurologic conditions

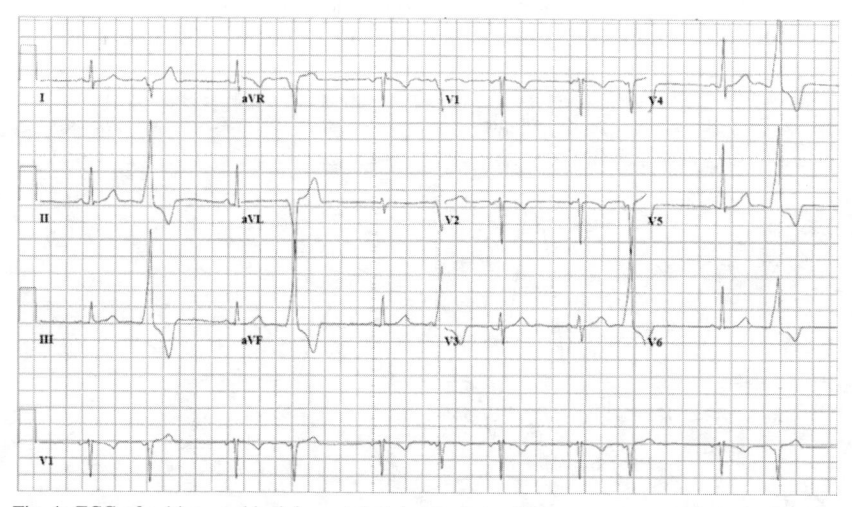

Fig 4. ECG of a 14-year-old adolescent that demonstrates frequent premature ventricular beats.

such as subarachnoid hemorrhage). Up to 90% of patients with HCM have some abnormal resting ECG readings,[4] often either ST-segment abnormalities or T-wave changes (Fig 6). Whereas infarction and ischemia are uncommon in adolescents, the term "early repolarization" is applied when it is associated with ST elevation, and it is most easily appreciated in the anterior and midprecordial leads (V2-V4) (Fig 7). The term is a misnomer (because repolarization normally begins before depolarization ends), and the associated elevation of the ST segment may be attributable to the normal age-dependent changes of ST-segment potentials. It can especially mimic changes that are seen in pericarditis. J-point elevation attributable to early repolarization often disappears with exercise. Table 1 summarizes common ECG features in myocardial ischemia or injury, pericarditis, and early repolarization.

Pericarditis is the most common cause of ST-segment elevation in children other than early repolarization (Fig 8).[5] Initially, the ST segment is elevated with a normal T wave, followed by normalization of the ST-segment and T-wave inversion. PR segment depression may also be seen. Usually, findings differ from ischemic changes because they involve all leads.[6] Myocarditis can result in ST-segment deviation or conduction abnormalities but most commonly presents with flattened or inverted T waves and low-voltage QRS patterns (<0.5 mV QRS amplitude in the limb leads and <1.0 mV in the precordial leads).[2] Fulminant myocarditis, the more hemodynamically severe form of the acute disease, often causes ventricular ectopy and tachycardia.

Myocardial ischemia is rarely seen in the adolescent population. It can occur in the setting of congenital abnormalities of the coronary arteries (Fig 9), as part of the sequelae of previous cardiac surgery or Kawasaki disease, in premature coronary atherosclerosis in patients with familial hypercholesterolemia, as late sequelae in adolescents after a heart transplant, or with the use of anabolic steroids or cocaine. Ischemic ECG changes manifest as ST-

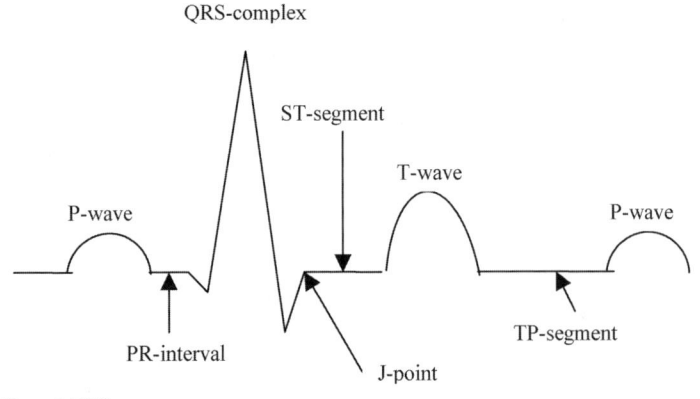

Fig 5. Normal ECG.

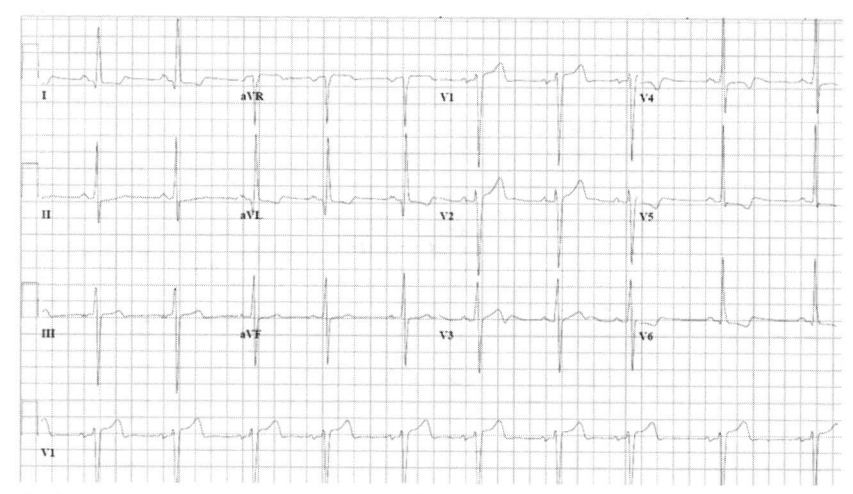

Fig 6. ECG in a 19-year-old male with HCM that demonstrates changes consistent with left-ventricular hypertrophy.

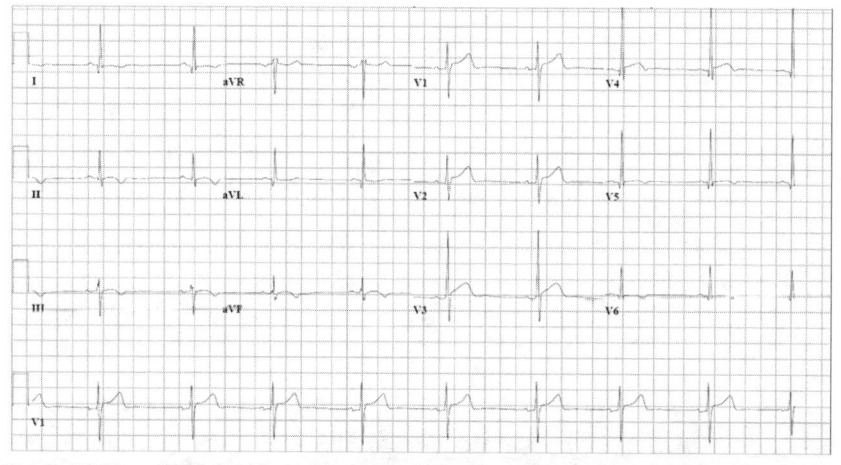

Fig 7. ECG in a 15-year-old boy with chest pain that demonstrates changes consistent with early repolarization. J-point elevation is appreciated in leads V1 to V4.

segment elevation or depression (a horizontal or downsloping ST segment is generally indicative of ischemia, and an upsloping ST segment is a poor indicator of ischemia) or T-wave inversion. The ST segment is compared with the TP segment at 60 to 80 milliseconds after the J point. ST depression of >2 mm or T-wave inversion in the lateral precordial leads (V5–V6) represents significant changes (Fig 10). Differential diagnosis includes subendocardial ischemia, hypertrophy with strain, or therapeutic digitalis use. T-wave inversion may be seen with ischemia, hyperventilation,[7] electrolyte abnormalities, intracranial pathology, and normal variants such as persistent juve-

Table 1
ECG features that differentiate early repolarization from pericarditis and myocardial ischemia or infarction

Feature	Myocardial Ischemia or Infarction	Pericarditis	Early Repolarization
PR depression	Rare	Frequent	Absent
Q waves	May be present	Absent	Absent
ST elevation	Convex and localized to area of related artery	Concave and widespread	Concave and localized (most prominent in leads V2–V4)
Reciprocal ST depression	May be present	Absent	Absent
T wave	Inverted when ST segments are still elevated	Inverted after ST segments have normalized	Normal or prominent
AV block, ventricular arrhythmias	Common	Absent	Absent

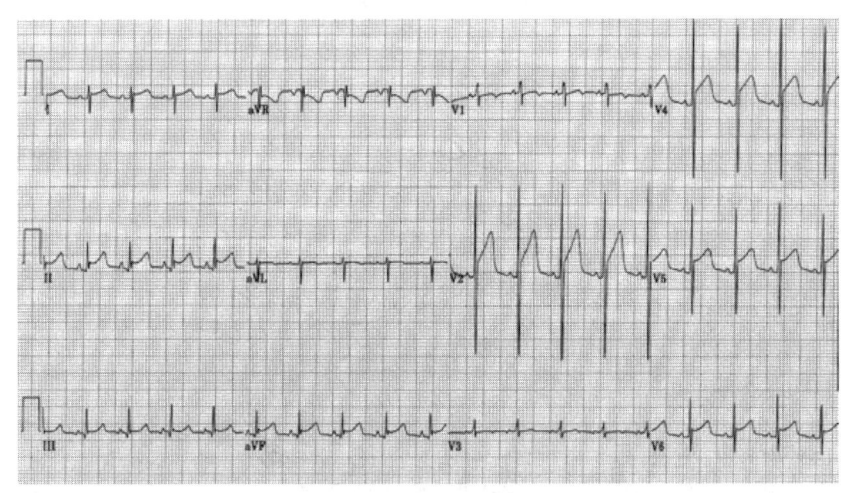

Fig 8. ECG in a 15-year-old girl with pericarditis. Widespread ST elevation can be seen.

nile pattern (T-wave inversion without ST elevation in leads V1–V3 with normal R wave progression) or benign T-wave inversion. Comparison to an old ECG can be of benefit.

Chest pain may be evaluated by either continuous or patient-activated ECG monitoring (see "Holter and event monitor"). However, on ambulatory ECG (AECG), a cardiac cause of chest pain is identified in <5% of pediatric patients,[8] and most AECG studies in pediatric patients have revealed no yield

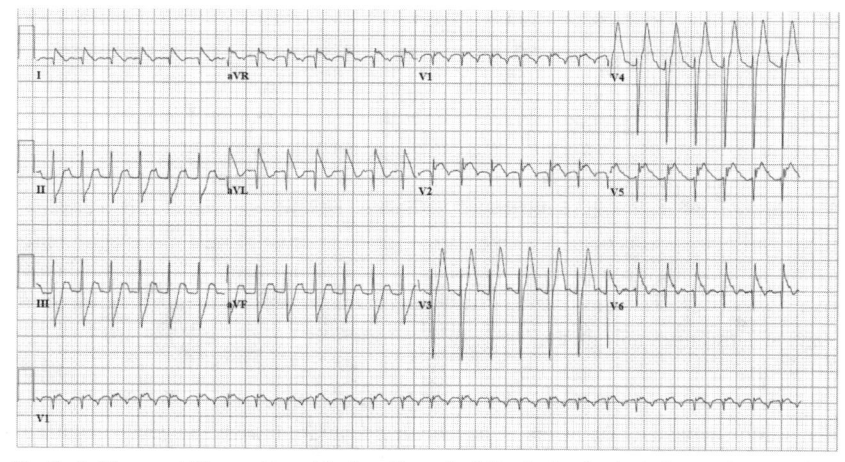

Fig 9. A 14-year-old boy, who suddenly collapsed while playing basketball, was found to have anomalous origin of left main coronary artery. ECG results demonstrate widespread ischemic changes.

in the evaluation of chest pain. The primary role of AECG monitoring in pediatric patients with chest pain may be to exclude rather than to diagnose a cardiac cause.

Evaluation of the QT Interval

A final interval of the ECG wave form is the QT interval. The QT segment represents the period between ventricular depolarization and repolarization, the length of which is influenced by ion movement through myocardial cell membrane channels. Abnormal ion movement can occur because of certain medications, autonomic states, and genetically determined channel abnormalities. The QT interval is measured from the beginning of the QRS complex to the end of the T wave in the lead with the longest interval and without a prominent U wave.[9] The best measurement of the QT interval is in leads II and V5.[10] The duration of the QT interval decreases with increasing heart

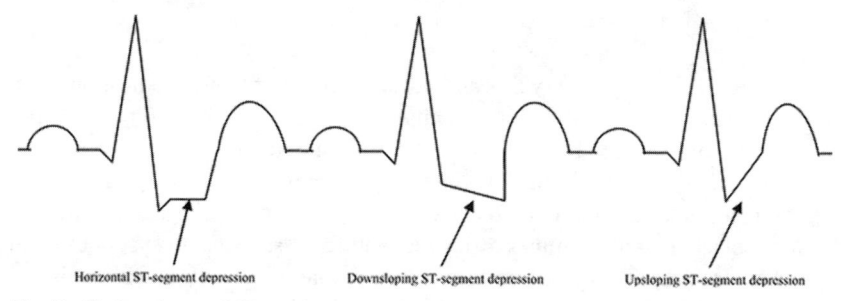

Fig 10. Various forms of ST-segment depression.

rates. Thus, the reference range for the QT interval is rate dependent. The QT interval duration varies from lead to lead and with age.[11] The corrected QT interval (QTc) relates the QT interval to heart rate in the formula developed by Bazett: QTc = QT/(R-R)½. The R-R interval preceding the measured QT interval is used for the calculation. Bazett's formula is not linear; it overcorrects for heart rates of <60 beats per minute and undercorrects at high rates.[10] A large recent study showed that the 98th percentile for the QTc (averaged across all age groups) was 449 milliseconds for men and 460 milliseconds for women.[12] For children aged 10 to 19 years, the upper limit of normal was 448 milliseconds for boys and 457 milliseconds for girls. For subjects aged 20 to 29 years, the upper limit was 436 milliseconds for men and 454 milliseconds for women.

The length of the QTc interval has been associated with the risk of sudden death after myocardial infarction and LQTS (Fig 11).[13] Familial LQTS is characterized by an abnormally prolonged QTc interval associated with T-wave abnormalities and ventricular arrhythmias (polymorphic VT and torsade de pointes). Patients typically present with syncope, seizures, or sudden death, which is often triggered by physical or emotional stress or loud noise. Disorders are inherited as an autosomal dominant pattern with variable penetrance (Romano-Ward syndrome) or, less frequently, as an autosomal recessive pattern (Jervell-Lange-Nielsen syndrome), which is also associated with deafness.[14] Sporadic cases without a known family history have also been described. Mutations in the genes that encode ion-channel proteins which control repolarization have been identified as underlying causes. The diagnosis is made by using a scoring system that combines data obtained from clinical and family histories and ECG results.[15] Serial ECGs provide the greatest opportunity for making an accurate diagnosis, because there is variability in the QT interval.[16] In ~25% of genetically proven cases, the QT interval actually falls into the reference range.[17] Exercise testing is also used to evaluate the absolute changes of the QT interval (normally, the QT interval shortens with exercise because of increased heart rate; however, it can abnormally lengthen). Available genetic testing is believed to currently identify ~70% to 75% of the mutations that cause LQTS.[10] When the question of LQTS is raised for an adolescent, first-degree relatives should also be screened.

Prolongation of the QT interval is an undesired effect of many medications and, in the context of a patient with congenital prolongation of the QT interval, can lead to life-threatening arrhythmias. There are a number of drugs (especially in combination) that prolong the QT interval (typically class 1A antiarrhythmic agents, macrolide and fluoroquinolone antibiotics, antimalarial agents, antifungal agents, selected antihistamines, tricyclic antidepressants, antipsychotics, and opioid analgesics). They must be used with caution in individuals with a history suggestive of LQTS, such as syncope or a family history of syncope, deafness,

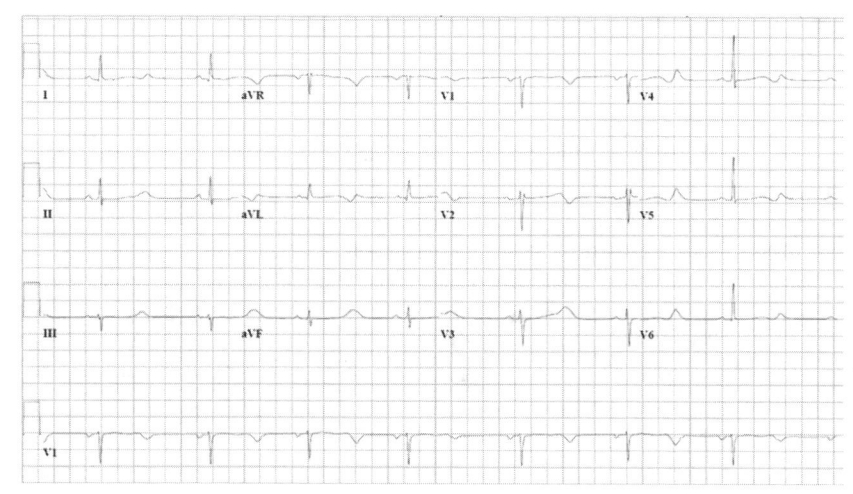

Fig 11. Prolonged QT interval. The QTc measures ~630 milliseconds.

or sudden death. Factors that predispose to development of torsade de pointes include bradycardia, hypokalemia, and hypomagnesemia. Serial ECGs are commonly used to monitor potential cardiac effects of certain psychotropic medications.[18] Adolescents who receive tricyclic antidepressants or antipsychotic/neuroleptic medications should be monitored for ECG changes (PR >200 milliseconds, QRS >120 milliseconds, QTc >460 milliseconds), in which case alternative therapy may need to be considered along with additional evaluation by a pediatric cardiologist. A follow-up ECG after therapeutic levels are reached should be obtained.

Use of ECG in Sports Participants' Screening

The ECG has relatively low specificity as a screening test in athletic populations, largely because of the high frequency of ECG alterations associated with the normal physiologic adaptations of the trained athlete's heart.[19] Under current recommendations, the AHA panel does not recommend the routine use of tests such as the 12-lead ECG or echocardiography in the context of mass, universal screening. This view is based on the substantial size of the athlete cohort to be screened, the relatively low prevalence of cardiovascular conditions responsible for sports-related deaths, the limited resources presently available for allocation, and, in particular, the absence of a physician-examiner cadre prepared and available to perform and interpret these examinations.

HOLTER AND EVENT MONITORING

Holter, or AECG, monitoring in the adolescent patient is indicated for evaluation of symptoms that may be arrhythmia related, risk assessment in patients with cardiovascular disease (with or without symptoms of an arrhythmia), and evaluation of cardiac rhythm after an intervention such as drug therapy or device implantation.

In adolescents with frequent symptoms that are possibly related to an arrhythmia such as palpitations, presyncope, syncope, dizziness, or chest pain, an AECG is an excellent tool for helping to correlate an arrhythmia with symptoms.[20] In contrast to the standard 12-lead ECG, which captures readings of a brief period of time (a few seconds), the ambulatory monitor records the cardiac rhythm over a prolonged period of time, usually 24 to 48 hours. It is an ideal test for patients with frequent (at least daily) arrhythmias and provides information on the frequency of occurrence, related symptoms, and potential exacerbating factors. An activity diary can aid in correlating symptoms to ECG findings. Between 25% and 50% of patients will have complaints of symptoms during the time they wear a Holter monitor. Of these patients, 2% to 15% will have a causal arrhythmia.[20,21] The second type of ambulatory monitoring is the event recorder. There are multiple technologies available. They can be broadly categorized as event recorders, loop recorders, or implantable long-term recorders. The event recorder typically records the electrogram on a continuous tape. Only the last 30 to 90 seconds are available for playback. When symptoms occur, the patient can stop the tape by pressing a button and transmit the information on the tape via telephone. This type of testing is best ordered for relatively infrequent symptoms that have been difficult to document. This monitor is carried for an extended period of time (usually several weeks) until a symptomatic episode is captured. More sophisticated loop devices can store presymptomatic, symptomatic, and postsymptomatic arrhythmia readings for a period of several minutes when activated. The diagnostic yield of such recorders is up to 60% in individuals with intermittent symptoms. The third option is an implantable rhythm monitor, which is a tiny microprocessor-based device placed under the skin that has the ability to record a patient's ECG for weeks to months. The information can be downloaded periodically and reviewed. This type of device is usually ordered and implanted by electrophysiologists.

A patient-activated recorder is generally recommended for the evaluation of palpitations, because of the paroxysmal nature of the symptom. An arrhythmia, usually supraventricular tachycardia, has been reported to correlate with palpitation in 10% to 15% of young patients, whereas ventricular ectopy or bradycardia is demonstrated in another 2% to 5%. Sinus tachycardia is identified in nearly 50% of young patients with symptoms of palpitation during ambulatory monitoring, whereas 30% to 40% of patients have no symptoms during monitoring.[20] One of the primary uses of AECG monitoring in adolescents is to exclude an arrhythmia as the cause of palpitation. The intermittent nature of symptoms results in a low efficacy of 24 to 48 hours of continuous ECG monitoring; conversely, temporary patient incapacitation usually precludes patient-activated recording. Continuous ECG monitoring is primarily indicated for pediatric patients with exertional symptoms or those with known heart disease, in whom the presence and significance of an arrhythmia may be increased.

AECG monitoring is commonly used in the periodic evaluation of pediatric patients with heart disease (Fig 12) with or without symptoms of an arrhythmia. The rationale for this testing is the evolution of disease processes (such as LQTS or HCM), growth of patients and the need to adjust medication dosages, and the progressive onset of late arrhythmias after surgery for congenital heart defects. The use of AECG monitoring for periodic evaluation of patients with previous surgical treatment of congenital heart disease must be based on consideration of the type of defect, ventricular function, and risk of late postoperative arrhythmias. For example, uncomplicated repairs of atrial or ventricular septal defects are associated with a low incidence of late postoperative arrhythmias. Complex repairs or those with residual hemodynamic abnormalities have a higher incidence of late-onset atrial and ventricular arrhythmias. Although the significance of arrhythmias in these patients remains controversial, high-grade ambulatory ventricular ectopy associated with ventricular dysfunction does seem to identify patients who are at an increased risk of late sudden death. Complex arrhythmias detected in these patients by AECG may indicate the need for additional investigation or intervention, even in the absence of overt symptoms.

Periodic AECG monitoring for young patients with HCM, dilated cardiomyopathies, or LQTS is recommended because of the progression of these diseases and the need to adjust medication doses with growth. The risk of sudden death with

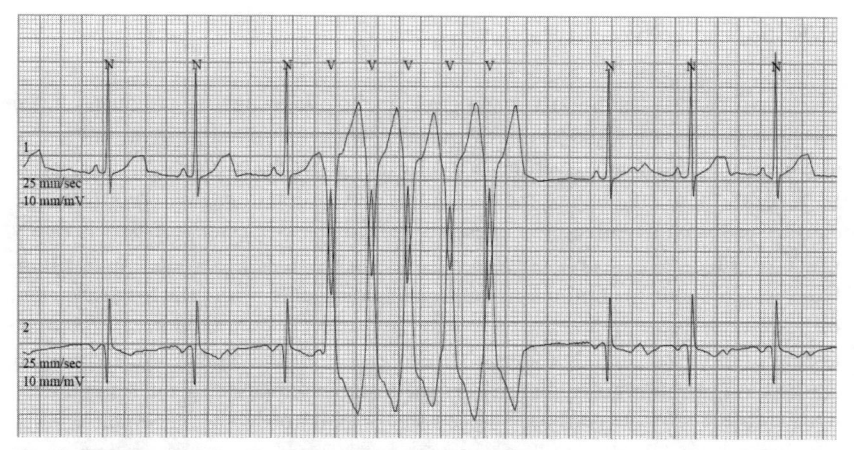

Fig 12. Holter monitoring of a 13-year-old adolescent with history of myocarditis, VT, and status post implantable cardioverter defibrillator shows recurrent VT.

these diseases is much greater in pediatric patients than adults, with sudden death as the first symptom occurring in 9% to 15% of patients.[22,23] One primary role of AECG monitoring is to identify occult arrhythmias, which may indicate the need for reevaluation of therapy in an asymptomatic patient. However, the absence of an arrhythmia during monitoring does not necessarily indicate a low risk of sudden death. AECG monitoring plays a limited role in establishing a diagnosis of LQTS in patients with borderline QT prolongation.

AECG monitoring may be used to identify asymptomatic patients with congenital complete AV block who are at increased risk for sudden arrhythmic events and, thus, may benefit from prophylactic pacemaker implantation. Routine AECG evaluation of asymptomatic patients with preexcitation syndromes (WPW) has not been demonstrated to define patients who are at risk for sudden arrhythmic death.

Arrhythmias have become increasingly recognized in young patients with a number of diverse medical conditions including Duchenne or Becker muscular dystrophy, myotonic dystrophy and those who are survivors of childhood malignancies. AECG monitoring may be indicated for these patients in the presence of symptoms compatible with an arrhythmia because of the potential for both ventricular arrhythmias and progressive conduction system disease.

AECG monitoring is useful for evaluating both beneficial and potentially adverse responses to pharmacologic therapy in pediatric patients. Additional indications for AECG monitoring include the evaluation of symptoms in patients with pacemakers or after radio-frequency catheter ablation or heart surgery, particularly when complicated by transient AV block. AECG monitoring is also indicated for the evaluation of cardiac rhythm after treatment of incessant tachyarrhythmias, which have been associated with progressive ventricular dysfunction.

STRESS TESTING

Reasons for stress testing in young people include investigating exercise-related symptoms, evaluating the stress of exercise on known cardiac conditions, and assessing the effectiveness of medications (eg, β-blockade effect on heart rate). In general, these studies are most appropriately ordered and supervised by the cardiologist with expertise in adolescent heart disease. Exercise testing is rarely needed to look for occult coronary obstructions in the pediatric population. Exercise capacity is diminished in some adolescents with heart disease, and measurement is often useful in evaluating subjective limitations.[24] Exercise testing of children and adolescents has a very low risk compared with testing of adults. Complications of pediatric exercise testing are extremely infrequent, even when testing is performed on populations of children with congenital cardiac defects and arrhythmias. Indications for exercise stress testing have been published in specific guidelines.[24,25]

Several different methods of stress testing are available, including treadmill or bicycle exercise with ECG monitoring, imaging by echocardiography during or just after exercise, or pharmacologic simulation of stress (eg, using dobutamine infusion) with imaging performed by echocardiographic or nuclear methods. Treadmill protocols are relatively simple for the patient, simulate typical activities in which they engage (representing a more physiologic stress), and provide important information about peak endurance, respiratory health, overall fitness, blood pressure response, and cardiac electrical activity. However, confounders may include lack of cooperation, poor coordination, or unfamiliarity with the procedure, especially in younger patients. Stress tests should be ordered in consideration of the pretest probability of the presence of a specific disease process, because sensitivity and specificity will need to be interpreted in this context.

Although chest pain is common in children and adolescents, the history and physical examination are generally adequate to exclude serious pathology and provide reassurance to the patient and family. Noncardiac chest pain is usually described as a brief stabbing or shooting pain that occurs with or without exercise. Pleuritic pain is common. Typical etiologies include gastroesophageal reflux, exercise-induced reactive airways disease, costochondritis, or anxiety. Routine use of exercise testing for evaluation of chest pain in children and adolescents is not required. Exercise testing is appropriate for evaluation of the uncommon child with chest pain that is typical of angina by description and consistently related to exercise. Exercise-induced bronchospasm is best identified by pulmonary function tests.

Exercise testing is an important component of the evaluation of adolescents who have unexplained syncope related to physical exertion. Features of syncope that suggest a potentially life-threatening cardiac event include an abrupt loss of consciousness (as opposed to a prodrome or aura), injury on impact (as opposed to a gradual "slump"), and syncope related to physical activity. Evaluation for possible arrhythmia, left-ventricular outflow obstruction, and cardiomyopathy is appropriate. Neurally mediated hypotension (NMH) may rarely manifest primarily as exercise-induced syncope, most often with symptoms that occur immediately after cessation of the activity.

Premature atrial contractions are common and benign in young persons. Exercise test evaluation of premature atrial contractions in adolescents is not required. Exercise testing helps in evaluation of selected cases in which the history suggests an exercise-related tachycardia. The majority of children with supraventricular tachycardia, however, will not have exercise-induced tachycardia.

Isolated premature ventricular depolarizations in asymptomatic children and adolescents usually disappear with the higher heart rates associated with exercise.

It is not necessary to perform formal laboratory testing to demonstrate this result. Exercise testing is often of value in diagnosing VT and assessing the efficacy of treatment. VT with exercise is often observed in children with no structural heart abnormality and in children with myocarditis, cardiomyopathy, or a congenital cardiac malformation. Arrhythmogenic right-ventricular dysplasia is an inherited cardiomyopathy particularly related to the development of VT with exercise. Measurement of shortening or prolongation of the QTc to exercise has been used as an adjunct in the diagnosis of LQTS.

TILT-TABLE TESTING

Tilt-table testing is used primarily to diagnose or confirm suspicion of NMH in patients with syncope or near syncope. The test, although relatively simple to perform, is somewhat uncomfortable for the patient and, thus, is usually reserved for situations in which the diagnosis is unclear from history and physical examination alone or in which response to empiric therapy has been limited. Although protocols used in performing tilt-table testing vary among centers, most laboratories tilt patients for 15 to 45 minutes at an angle of 60° to 85°. After baseline parameters are measured, the patient is secured to a table and tilted. Normally, individuals compensate for such a tilt by increasing both α- and β-adrenergic tone as a result of baroreceptor stimulation, thus compensating for the decrease in venous return. In susceptible individuals, these compensatory mechanisms eventually collapse, and venous return is never completely compensated. As a result, sympathetic tone increases, which produces vigorous ventricular contractions of a relatively empty heart. This results in recruitment of cardiac C fibers, which causes stimulation of the medullary vasodepressor region. The result is a sudden withdrawal of sympathetic tone, a sudden increase in vagal tone, vasodilation, and syncope. If the test result is negative, the table is lowered in the original horizontal position, an intravenous infusion of isoproterenol is started and the dose is adjusted to increase the baseline heart rate to >20%. The tilt-table test is repeated for 15 to 20 minutes. Syncopal episodes have been shown to be preceded by a catecholamine surge. The addition of isoproterenol increases the sensitivity of the tilt-table test.

Questions about the sensitivity, specificity, diagnostic yield, and day-to-day reproducibility of tilt-table testing have been raised in the most recent AHA and American College of Cardiology Foundation scientific statement on the evaluation of syncope.[26] The reported sensitivity and specificity of tilt-table testing depend on the technique used. Sensitivity ranges from 26% to 80%, and specificity is ~90%. In their statement, the AHA and American College of Cardiology Foundation argue that in patients with a negative evaluation (ie, no evidence of ischemia and a structurally normal heart), the pretest probability that the diagnosis is neurocardiogenic syncope is high; hence, head-up tilt-table testing contributes little to establishing the diagnosis.

Table 2
Response patterns to tilt-table testing

Pattern	Blood Pressure	Pulse	Response
Normal	No change or slight increase	No change or slight increase	No symptoms
NMH	Rapid decrease	Decrease	Presyncope/syncope
POTS	No change or decrease	Increase	Presyncope
Dysautonomia	Gradual decrease	No change or increase	Presyncope/syncope
Psychogenic	No change or slight increase	No change or slight increase	Presyncope/syncope

Adapted from the results of Feinberg and Layne-Davies.[37]

Syncope is common in adolescents, with up to 47% of college students reporting fainting episodes[27] Syncope is a disabling condition that requires attention, but it is generally not life-threatening. It can be frightening to patients, families, and primary care providers. If cardiac or neurologic abnormalities are not apparent after a thorough history and physical examination have been performed, and blood, ECG, and echocardiogram results are normal, tilt-table testing is often used as an aid in establishing the diagnosis of NMH and postural orthostatic tachycardia syndrome (POTS).

NMH is defined by a decrease in systolic blood pressure of >25 mm Hg (compared with the blood pressure measured when the person lies flat) during standing or upright tilt-table testing.[28] POTS is defined by an exaggerated increase in heart rate while the patient stands. A healthy teenager usually has a slight increase in heart rate by ~10 to 15 beats per minute within the first 10 minutes of standing. POTS is considered present if the heart rate increases >30 beats per minute (or if it reaches 120 beats per minute or higher) over the first 10 minutes of standing.[29] Some patients with POTS in the first 10 minutes of standing or tilt testing will go on to develop NMH if the test is continued. Different response patterns to the tilt-table test in normal individuals and in those with NMH, POTS, dysautonomia, and psychogenic syncope are listed in Table 2.

ECHOCARDIOGRAPHY

Echocardiography is the primary tool of the cardiologist for diagnosing structural heart disease, and its results are highly accurate when it is performed and interpreted by experienced laboratory professionals. However, screening for heart disease, especially in the adolescent and young adult, is still more appropriately performed by carefully studying a patient's history and physical examination results. The more important role for echocardiography in an adolescent is in fully characterizing a cardiac lesion once an abnormality is suspected. It also provides essential information concerning the natural history of the abnormality and responses to medical and surgical management. A transthoracic echocardio-

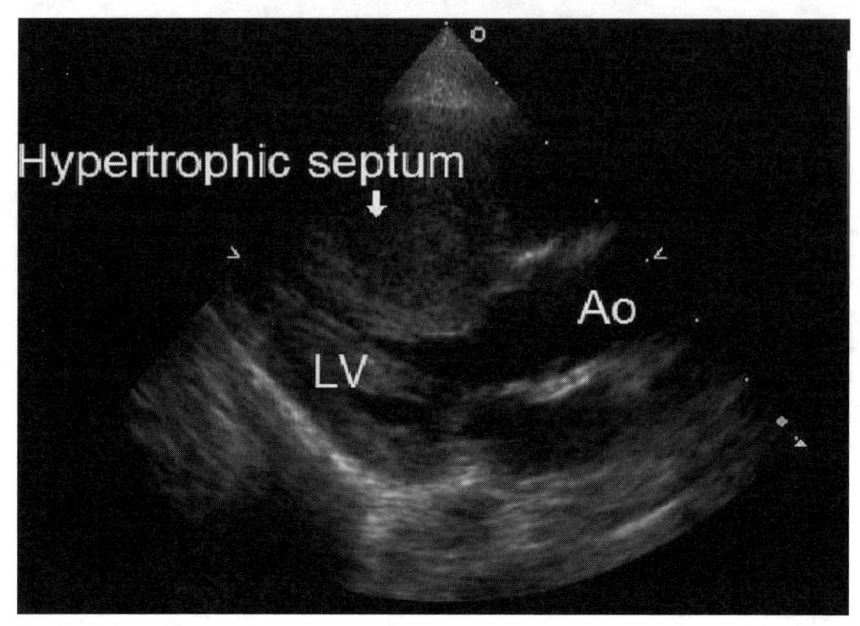

Fig 13. Echocardiogram of a 19-year-old young adult who demonstrates HCM. Ao indicates aorta; LV, left ventricle.

gram is a reliable and versatile tool for the assessment of cardiac structure, function, and pathophysiology. It is associated with little, if any, patient discomfort and no risks. Because it depends on obtaining satisfactory examining windows from the body surface to the cardiovascular structures, there may be limitations to its use. In the obese adolescent, the interposition of adipose tissue between body surface and the heart can limit image quality, and complete examination may not be possible. Echocardiographic contrast agents (administered through a peripheral access line) that can pass through the pulmonary circulation and opacify the left heart have been developed and become a useful aid in the evaluation of obese patients. For specific indications (eg, evaluation for endocarditis or intracardiac thrombus), transesophageal echocardiography is an excellent tool for additional assessment. The echocardiographic transducer is mounted on a flexible endoscope and passed into the esophagus and stomach. However, this technique is invasive and requires sedation and intubation.

Indications for the performance of an adolescent echocardiogram span a wide range of symptoms and signs, including exercise-induced chest pain or syncope, murmurs, respiratory distress, abnormal arterial pulses, and cardiomegaly, which may suggest structural heart disease. An echocardiogram is indicated for the evaluation of acquired heart diseases in children, including rheumatic fever and carditis, infective endocarditis, HIV infection, myocarditis, pericarditis, Kawasaki disease (for follow-up), all forms of cardiomyopathies (Fig 13), systemic lupus erythematosus, renal disease, and connective-tissue diseases with known cardiovascular manifestations (Marfan syndrome, Loeys-Dietz syndrome). Patients receiving anthracycline or other cardiotoxic agents should have baseline and reevaluation follow-up studies. Pediatric echocardiography is indicated in the assessment of potential cardiac or cardiopulmonary transplant donors and transplant recipients. Echocardiography has been recommended for all children who have been newly diagnosed with systemic hypertension.[30] Noncardiac disease states that affect the heart, such as pulmonary hypertension, constitute an important indication for serial pediatric echocardiograms. Echocardiography may also be indicated for adolescents with thromboembolic events (eg, sickle cell disease). Elevated right-ventricular and pulmonary artery pressure, as estimated by echo-Doppler evaluation of tricuspid regurgitation, correlates with increased mortality risk in patients with sickle cell disease.[31] Children with arrhythmias may have previously undiagnosed structural cardiac disease such as congenitally corrected transposition, Ebstein's anomaly of the tricuspid valve, or cardiomyopathy, which may be associated with subtle clinical findings and are best evaluated by using echocardiography. Sustained arrhythmias or antiarrhythmic medications may lead to functional impairment of the heart that may only be detectable by echocardiography and have important implications for management. Practice guidelines for the clinical application of echocardiography have been published by the American College of Cardiology/AHA.[32–35]

Cardiovascular disease in the adolescent includes anomalies of cardiac anatomy, function, and rhythm. Although problems often present as an asymptomatic heart murmur, cardiac murmurs in this age group are more commonly functional than pathologic. The contribution of echocardiography to the evaluation of an asymptomatic patient with this finding on routine examination by an experienced clinician is limited. The use of a patient history and skilled physical examination are usually sufficient to distinguish functional from pathologic murmurs and are more cost-effective than referral for an echocardiogram.[36] However, in the presence of ambiguous clinical findings, echocardiography can demonstrate the presence or absence of abnormalities such as an interatrial septal defect, bicuspid aortic valve, mildly obstructive subaortic stenosis, mitral valve prolapse, aortic aneurysm, or functionally occult cardiomyopathy.

RADIOLOGIC STUDIES

The chest radiograph is an important clinical tool in cardiovascular evaluation. In many cases heart disease is associated with cardiomegaly. A quantitative estimate of heart size may be obtained by determining the cardiothoracic ratio, which is calculated by dividing the maximal transverse diameter of the heart in the posteroanterior view by the width of the thoracic cavity. As a general rule, the heart is enlarged if the cardiothoracic ratio is >0.5. Although the cardiothoracic ratio is useful in the detection of cardiomegaly in cases of left-ventricular

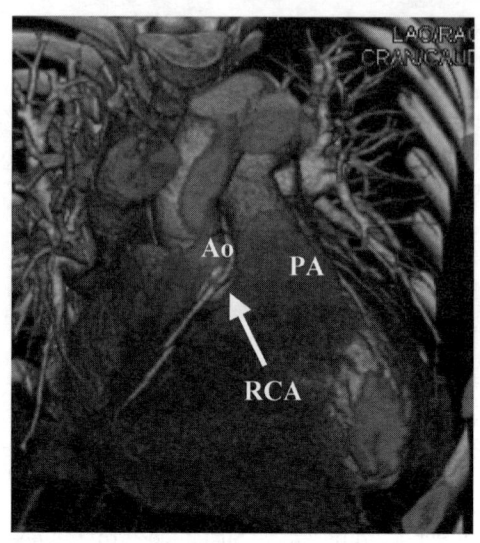

Fig 14. Cardiac CT in an adolescent boy who demonstrates anomalous origin of the right coronary artery (RCA) from the left coronary sinus and traversing between the aorta (Ao) and pulmonary artery (PA).

enlargement or pericardial effusion, it is not as sensitive in the assessment of right-ventricular enlargement.

Cardiovascular MRI is a well-established diagnostic imaging technique with emerging roles in the evaluation of cardiovascular disease. Its ability to acquire high-resolution images in virtually any plane, to make accurate measurements of blood velocity flow and cardiac volumes, to perform noninvasive angiography, and to assess myocardial mechanics and perfusion, all in the absence of ionizing radiation, promotes its versatility. Indications include, but are not limited to, evaluation of congenital heart disease, evaluation of aortic disease, assessment of intrinsic nonischemic myocardial disease, assessment of ischemic heart disease, assessment of valvular heart disease, evaluation of the pericardium, evaluation of cardiac masses, and assessment of pulmonary arteries. Contraindications to the use of this technique are mainly related to electrically, magnetically, or mechanically active implants in a patient's body.

Indications for cardiovascular CT have rapidly expanded over the last years, mainly secondary to technical improvements that allow for faster scanning with increased special resolution. Clinical indications range from assessment of the great vessels to noninvasive imaging of the coronary arteries (Fig 14). Cardiac CT is a noninvasive alternative test to cardiac catheterization. Current technologies include electron-beam CT and multiple-detector CT . Electron-beam CT involves the use of a rapidly oscillating electron beam reflected onto a stationary target. It has a high temporal resolution, and the slice thickness is 1.5 to 3.0 mm, covering the entire heart in 1 or 2 breath-hold periods. Multiple-detector CT involves the use of a mechanically rotated x-ray tube at high speed. This type of scanner is used for noncardiac and cardiac imaging with a minimal slice thickness of 0.75 mm to 1.0 mm, covering the entire heart in a single breath-hold. Clinical indications include coronary artery assessment (calcium scoring, CT angiography), cardiac chamber assessment, evaluation of the great vessels, evaluation of congenital heart disease, and assessment of pericardial disease. The downside of this technique remains the need to use radiation. Whereas the average risk for radiation-induced cancer in the general population is estimated at 5% per 1 Sv, in children and adolescents the risk is predicted to be up to 2 to 3 times higher than that in adults (as high as 15% per 1 Sv).[37] The typical effective radiation dose for a cardiac CT angiography is estimated to be in the order of 10 to 25 mSv. In comparison, the typical effective radiation dose for a chest radiograph equals 0.1 to 0.2 mSv.[38]

Positron-emitting tracers (PETs) can be used to study myocardial blood flow, glucose and fatty acid metabolism, and oxygen consumption. The PET scan is an established method for the evaluation of myocardial viability in adults with ischemic heart disease. In pediatrics, the application of PETs has been limited. Potential applications include the evaluation of ischemic changes that may occur in different diseases of the coronary arteries (congenital anomalies, Kawasaki disease, and certain postoperative repairs such as the arterial switch procedure).

CARDIAC CATHETERIZATION AND ELECTROPHYSIOLOGY STUDY

The development of excellent noninvasive techniques has allowed many patients' heart disease to be diagnosed and treated. Nevertheless, cardiac catheterization remains a vital tool in the evaluation and treatment of adolescents with congenital or acquired heart disease. Cardiac catheterization before cardiac surgery is indicated when a full anatomic diagnosis or necessary hemodynamic measurements cannot be made by noninvasive tests or when the clinical picture is inconsistent with the patient's presumptive diagnosis. Cardiac catheterization is used to evaluate patients before heart transplantation and perform surveillance biopsies to evaluate for subclinical rejection after cardiac transplantation. Cardiac biopsy obtained at catheterization is used to diagnose myocarditis. Furthermore, during cardiac catheterization patients can be evaluated for pulmonary hypertension, and their response to drug therapy can be assessed. Detailed indications for specific cardiac lesions are beyond the scope of this review. The field of therapeutic cardiac catheterization continues to expand. Percutaneous device closures of atrial septal defect, patent foramen ovale, patent ductus arteriosus, or stent enlargement of coarctation of the aorta are only a few examples. Overall, the risk associated with this technique is low. It should also be kept in mind that cardiac catheterizations are among the radiologic procedures with the highest patient radiation dose, which remains a source of great concern in the pediatric population. For an average diagnostic cardiac catheterization, a median effective radiation dose of 4.6 mSv has been found. Therapeutic procedures result in a higher median effective radiation dose of 6.0 mSv.[39]

The electrophysiology study is a specialized form of cardiac catheterization that can be helpful in evaluating a broad spectrum of cardiac arrhythmias. It can assess the function of the sinus node, the AV node, and the His-Purkinje system. It can also determine the mechanism and characteristics of tachyarrhythmias and locate reentrant circuits (accessory pathways). Finally, it can evaluate the efficacy of antiarrhythmic medication and devices. During the procedure, multiple electrodes are placed in the heart, which record the electrical signals from the atria, AV node, and ventricles. Pacing from localized areas within the heart is used to induce the arrhythmia to be studied. If an amenable tachycardia is identified, an ablation procedure can be performed, thus interrupting the aberrant electrical pathways. Ablation techniques use heat (radio frequency) or cold (cryoablation) to produce thermal damage to the myocardial tissue. Procedures can be repeated for recurrences. Specific guidelines for intracardiac electrophysiological and catheter ablation procedures have been published.[40]

REFERENCES

1. Schlant RC, Adolph RJ, DiMarco JP, et al. Guidelines for electrocardiography: a report of the American College of Cardiology/American Heart Association Task Force on Assessment of Diagnostic and Therapeutic Cardiovascular Procedures (Committee on Electrocardiography). *Circulation.* 1992;85(3):1221–1228
2. Kadish AH, Buxton AE, Kennedy HL, et al. ACC/AHA clinical competence statement on electrocardiography and ambulatory electrocardiography: a report of the American College of Cardiology/American Heart Association/American College of Physicians-American Society of Internal Medicine Task Force on Clinical Competence (ACC/AHA Committee to Develop a Clinical Competence Statement on Electrocardiography and Ambulatory Electrocardiography). *Circulation.* 2001;104(25):3169–3178
3. Estes MNA. Diagnostic techniques. In: Lewis RP, O'Gara PT, Hirsch G, eds. *Adult Clinical Cardiology Self-assessment Program 6.* Bethesda, MD: American College of Cardiology Foundation; 2005:15.11–15.23
4. Maron BJ. The electrocardiogram as a diagnostic tool for hypertrophic cardiomyopathy: revisited. *Ann Noninvasive Electrocardiol.* 2001;6(4):277–279
5. Van Hare GF, Dubin A. The normal electrocardiogram. In: Allen HD, Gutgesell HP, Clark EB, Driscoll DJ, eds. *Moss and Adams' Heart Disease in Infants, Children, and Adolescents.* 6th ed. Philadelphia, PA: Lippincott, Williams & Wilkins; 2001:425–442
6. Spodick DH. Electrocardiogram in acute pericarditis. *Am J Cardiol.* 1974;33(4):470–474
7. Wasserburger RH, Alt WJ, Lloyd CJ. The normal RS-T segment elevation variant. *Am J Cardiol.* 1961;8(2):184–192
8. Selbst SM, Ruddy RM, Clark BJ, Henretig FM, Santulli T Jr. Pediatric chest pain: a prospective study. *Pediatrics.* 1988;82(3):319–323
9. Bednar MM, Harrigan EP, Anziano RJ, Camm AJ, Ruskin JN. The QT interval. *Prog Cardiovasc Dis.* 2001;43(suppl I):1–45

10. Vetter V. Clues or miscues? how to make the right interpretation and correctly diagnose long-QT syndrome. *Circulation.* 2007;115(20):2595-2598
11. Davignon A, Rautaharju PM, Boisselle E, Soumis F, Megelas M, Choquette A. Normal ECG standards for infants and children. *Pediatr Cardiol.* 1980;1:123-131
12. Mason JW, Ramseth DJ, Chanter DO, Moon TE, Goodman DB, Mendzelevski B. Electrocardiographic reference ranges derived from 79,743 ambulatory subjects. *J Electrocardiol.* 2007;40(3): 228-234
13. Moss AJ. Measurement of the QT interval and the risk associated with QTc interval prolongation: a review. *Am J Cardiol.* 1993;72(6):23B-25B
14. Camm AJ, Janse MJ, Roden DM, Rosen MR, Cinca J, Cobbe SM. Congenital and acquired long QT syndrome. *Eur Heart J.* 2000;21(15):1232-1237
15. Schwartz PJ, Moss AJ, Vincent GM, Crampton RS. Diagnostic criteria for the long QT syndrome: an update. *Circulation.* 1993;88(2):782-784
16. Goldenberg I, Matthew I, Moss AJ, et al. Corrected QT variability in serial electrograms in long QT syndrome: the importance of the maximum corrected QT for risk stratification. *J Am Coll Cardiol.* 2006;48(5):1047-1052
17. Tester DJ, Will ML, Haglund CM, Ackerman MJ. Effect of clinical phenotype on yield of long QT syndrome genetic testing. *J Am Coll Cardiol.* 2006;47(4):764-768
18. Gutgesell H, Atkins D, Barst R, et al. Cardiovascular monitoring of children and adolescents receiving psychotropic drugs: a statement for healthcare professionals from the Committee on Congenital Cardiac Defects, Council on Cardiovascular Disease in the Young, American Heart Association. *Circulation.* 1999;99(7):979-982
19. Maron BJ, Thompson PD, Ackerman MJ, et al. Recommendations and considerations related to preparticipation screening for cardiovascular abnormalities in competitive athletes: 2007 update: a scientific statement from the American Heart Association Council on Nutrition, Physical Activity, and Metabolism: endorsed by the American College of Cardiology Foundation. *Circulation.* 2007;115(12):1643-1655
20. Crawford MH, Bernstein SJ, Deedwania PC, et al. ACC/AHA Guidelines for Ambulatory Electrocardiography: a report of the American College of Cardiology/American Heart Association Task Force on Practice Guidelines (Committee to Revise the Guidelines for Ambulatory Electrocardiography) developed in collaboration with the North American Society for Pacing and Electrophysiology. *J Am Coll Cardiol.* 1999;34(3):912-948
21. Watake J, Camm AJ. Holter and event recordings for arrhythmia detection. In: Zareba W, Maison-Blanche P, Locati E, eds. *Noninvasive Electrocardiography in Clinical Practice.* Armonk, NY: Futura Publishing Co, Inc; 2001:3-30
22. McKenna WJ, Franklin RC, Nihoyannopoulos P, Robinson KC, Deanfield JE. Arrhythmia and prognosis in infants, children and adolescents with hypertrophic cardiomyopathy. *J Am Coll Cardiol.* 1988;11(1):147-153
23. Garson A Jr, Dick M II, Fournier A, et al. The long QT syndrome in children: an international study of 287 patients. *Circulation.* 1993;87(6):1866-1872
24. Gibbons RJ, Balady GJ, Beasley JW, et al. ACC/AHA guidelines for exercise testing: a report of the American College of Cardiology/American Heart Association Task Force on Practice Guidelines (Committee on Exercise Testing). *J Am Coll Cardiol.* 1997;30(1):260-315
25. Paridon SM, Alpert BS, Boas SR, et al. AHA scientific statement on clinical stress testing in the pediatric age group: a statement from the American Heart Association Council on Cardiovascular Disease in the Young, Committee on Atherosclerosis, Hypertension, and Obesity in Youth. *Circulation.* 2006;113(15):1905-1920
26. Strickberger AS, Benson WD, Biaggioni I, et al. AHA/ACCF scientific statement on the evaluation of syncope. *J Am Coll Cardiol.* 2006;47(2):473-484
27. Feinberg AN, Lane-Davies A. Syncope in the adolescent. *Adolesc Med.* 2002;13(3):553-567
28. Rowe PC, Calkins H, DeBusk K, et al. Fludrocortisone acetate to treat neurally mediated hypotension in chronic fatigue syndrome: a randomized, controlled trial. *JAMA.* 2001;285(1):52-59
29. Grubb BP, Yousuf K, Kosinski DJ. The postural tachycardia syndrome: a concise guide to diagnosis and management. *J Cardiovasc Electrophysiol.* 2006;17(1):108-112

30. Falkner B, Daniels SR. Summary of the fourth report on the diagnosis, evaluation and treatment of high blood pressure in children and adolescent. *Hypertension.* 2004;44(4):387–388
31. Gladwin MT, Sachdev V, Jison ML, et al. Pulmonary hypertension as a risk factor for death in patients with sickle cell disease. *N Engl J Med.* 2004;350(9):886–895
32. Cheitlin MD, Alpert JS, Armstrong WF, et al. ACC/AHA guidelines for the clinical application of echocardiography. *Circulation.* 1997;95(6):1686–1744
33. Cheitlin MD, Armstrong WF, Aurigemma GP, et al. ACC/AHA/ASE 2003 guideline update for the clinical application of echocardiography: summary article—a report of the American College of Cardiology/American Heart Association Task Force on Practice Guidelines (ACC/AHA/ASE Committee to Update the 1997 Guidelines for the Clinical Application of Echocardiography). *Circulation.* 2003;108(9):1146–1162
34. Ayres NA, Miller-Hance W, Fyfe DA, et al. Indications and guidelines for performance of transesophageal echocardiography in the patient with pediatric acquired or congenital heart disease: a report from the Task Force of the Pediatric Council of the American Society of Echocardiography. *J Am Soc Echocardiogr.* 2005;18(1):91–98
35. Bonow RO, Carabello BA, Kanu C, et al. ACC/AHA 2006 guidelines for the management of patients with valvular heart disease: a report of the American College of Cardiology/American Heart Association Task Force on Practice Guidelines (Writing Committee to Revise the 1998 Guidelines for the Management of Patients With Valvular Heart Disease). Developed in collaboration with the Society of Cardiovascular Anesthesiologists. Endorsed by the Society for Cardiovascular Angiography and Interventions and the Society of Thoracic Surgeons [published correction appears in *Circulation.* 2007;115(15):e409]. *Circulation.* 2006;114(5):e84–e231
36. Newburger JW, Rosenthal A, Williams RG, Fellows K, Miettinen OS. Noninvasive tests in the initial evaluation of heart murmurs in children. *N Engl J Med.* 1983;308(2):61–64
37. Hall EJ. Lessons we have learned from our children: cancer risks from diagnostic radiology. *Pediatr Radiol.* 2002;32(10):700–706
38. Hunold P, Vogt FM, Schmermund A, et al. Radiation exposure during cardiac CT: effective doses at multi-detector row CT and electron-beam CT. *Radiology.* 2003;226(1):145–152
39. Bacher K, Bogaert E, Lapere R, De Wolf D, Thierens H. Patient-specific dose and radiation risk estimation in pediatric cardiac catheterization. *Circulation.* 2005;111(1):83–89
40. Zipes DP, DiMarco JP, Gillette PC, et al. Guidelines for clinical intracardiac electrophysiological and catheter ablation procedures: a report of the American College of Cardiology/American Heart Association Task Force on Practice Guidelines (Committee on Clinical Intracardiac Electrophysiologic and Catheter Ablation Procedures), developed in collaboration with the North American Society of Pacing and Electrophysiology. *J Am Coll Cardiol.* 1995;26(2):555–573

Imaging in Adolescent Medicine

Renee Flax-Goldenberg, MD*

Division of Pediatric Radiology, Department of Radiology, Johns Hopkins Medical Institutions, Nelson Basement N-157, 600 North Wolfe Street, Baltimore, MD, 21287, USA

Choosing the best imaging study for some of the common clinical entities encountered in the adolescent population is challenging. In all cases, a thorough history and physical examination are the foundation for arriving at a concise differential diagnosis. The purpose of imaging should be to confirm or rule out suspected pathology that requires immediate intervention or to further narrow the differential and direct additional imaging investigation accordingly. The topics for this article include suspected appendicitis, severe headache, acute-onset chest pain, acute-onset scrotal pain, lower abdominal and pelvic pain in adolescent girls, and suspected nephrolithiasis.

SUSPECTED APPENDICITIS

Appendicitis is the most common acute condition of the abdomen that requires surgery in all patient populations.[1] Peak incidence is in the late teenage years and early 20s, with a male/female ratio of 3:2 in teenagers and young adults. The ratio equalizes by the time patients reach their mid-30s.

When a patient seeks medical attention with the classic complaint of diffuse periumbilical pain that localizes to the right-lower quadrant with history of fever, nausea, and anorexia and on examination there is right-lower-quadrant tenderness, a strong suspicion of appendicitis should exist. Unfortunately, this classic history occurs in only 50% to 60% of patients. Any combination of these symptoms may occur. The migration of pain is the most discriminating historical feature, with sensitivity and specificity of ~80%.

Imaging methods, such as graded compression color Doppler ultrasonography and computed tomography (CT), have become increasingly important for decreasing the morbidity and mortality rates that result from the disease. They are aimed at avoiding a misdiagnosis and facilitating earlier surgery.

---

*Corresponding author.
E-mail address: rflaxgo1@jhmi.edu (R. Flax-Goldenberg).

Copyright © 2008 American Academy of Pediatrics. All rights reserved. ISSN 1934-4287

The decision to obtain ultrasonography or CT imaging depends on institutional preference and available expertise.[2,3]

Advantages of ultrasonography include low cost; the lack of ionizing radiation or need for patient preparation; short acquisition time; potential for diagnosis of other causes of abdominal pain, particularly in the subset of women of childbearing age; and the ability to provide dynamic information through graded compression.[1] The main disadvantages are operator dependency and limitations that result from body habitus and patient cooperation. A positive ultrasonography finding greatly helps rule in the diagnosis of appendicitis. A negative ultrasonography finding, however, does not exclude appendicitis unless a normal appendix is confidently visualized, which is rare. Ultrasonography examination of the patient who is suspected to have appendicitis should include a thorough evaluation of both the abdomen and the pelvic organs. The use of high-frequency linear probes, graded compression, and the addition of color Doppler ultrasonography all increase the sensitivity of the examination.[3]

In experienced hands, ultrasonography has reported sensitivities of 75% to 90%, specificities of 86% to 100%, accuracies of 87% to 96%, positive predictive values of 91% to 94%, and negative predictive values of 89% to 97% for the diagnosis of acute appendicitis.[4-6]

A normal appendix is observed infrequently when using gray-scale ultrasonography, but it can be visualized as a blind-ended, tubular, compressible intestinal loop that is continuous with the cecum and has a diameter of <6 mm. Classic ultrasound findings of acute appendicitis include an aperistaltic, noncompressible, blind-ended loop of bowel that arises from the base of the cecum with an outer diameter of >6 mm, echogenic prominent pericecal fat (fat stranding), an appendicolith, and periappendiceal fluid collection.

Ultrasonographic examination is also useful for diagnosing alternate pathologies such as tuboovarian abscess, ovarian torsion, ovarian cyst, or mesenteric adenitis, especially in women of childbearing age. Endovaginal examination should be added for sexually active women with unremarkable transabdominal pelvic ultrasound findings. This is of particular importance because of the overlap in the symptoms of appendicitis with those of gynecologic disease in women in their childbearing years. In addition, the appendix may have a pelvic location, in which case it may be seen clearly on the endovaginal image when it is not evident on the transabdominal image.

Advantages of CT in the diagnosis of acute appendicitis include less operator dependency than ultrasonography; enhanced delineation of the extent of the disease in the case of perforated appendicitis; easier visualization of a retrocecal appendix; unchanged quality of imaging regardless of the presence of bowel gas, obesity, or severe abdominal pain; and the possibility of multiplanar retrospective data reconstruction. Disadvantages of CT include the higher cost, potential risks of contrast media, and ionizing radiation exposure, which is especially critical when imaging children and young adults.[2]

Helical CT has reported sensitivities of 90% to 100%, specificities of 91% to 99%, accuracies of 94% to 98%, positive predictive values of 92% to 98%, and negative predictive values of 95% to 100% for the diagnosis of acute appendicitis.[4,6]

A variety of techniques are being used at different institutions, and there is considerable controversy in the literature regarding whether to use oral, rectal, or intravenous contrast agents and the question of whether the area scanned should be limited.[5,6]

The most popular and conservative approach is to perform helical CT scanning of the entire abdomen and pelvis with intravenous and oral contrast material. Proponents of this technique believe that contrast-enhanced CT is essential for the diagnosis and staging of numerous inflammatory, ischemic, and neoplastic processes that may cause acute abdominal pain and may simulate appendicitis.[5,6]

Intravenous contrast material has been shown to aid in the diagnosis of appendicitis by permitting the identification of the inflamed appendix. This may be critical for patients with mild appendicitis and a paucity of mesenteric fat and for those with perforated appendicitis. Opacification of the terminal ileum and cecum with oral contrast material has been advocated for avoiding false-positive results, in which fluid-filled terminal ileal loops are misdiagnosed as distended, inflamed appendices. Moreover, opacification of the normal appendix serves to exclude appendicitis.[4] Some centers advocate the use of rectal contrast to facilitate opacification of the appendix.[6] CT should be performed with the lowest dose that allows the radiologist to provide the necessary diagnostic information.

Specific CT findings of appendicitis include enlargement of the appendix (>6 mm in outer diameter), enhancement of the appendiceal wall, lack of opacification in an enlarged appendix, fat stranding in the periappendiceal region, and the presence of an appendicolith within the appendix.

HEADACHES IN ADOLESCENTS

More than 50% of adolescents suffer from headaches. Most of them do not need any diagnostic imaging. After a detailed history and complete physical, including a thorough neurologic examination, it is usually possible to narrow down the differential diagnosis and identify which patients need additional diagnostic imaging.

Although most neuroimaging studies performed for headache in the pediatric and adolescent population demonstrate no abnormalities, there are certain temporal patterns, descriptions of the type of pain, and abnormalities on neurologic examination that warrant neuroimaging.[7,8]

The US Headache Consortium, the American College of Emergency Physicians, and the American College of Radiology have all conducted extensive studies of the literature to develop recommendations for neuroimaging for patients with headache.[8]

High priority for neuroimaging exists for patients with thunderclap headache, focal neurologic symptoms, headache with exertion, headache that awakens the patient, a chronic/progressive pattern, and papilledema or abnormal neurologic examination findings (ataxia, abnormal reflexes, etc).[8-10]

Nearly every life-threatening condition that could cause a headache can be seen on a noncontrast CT. This examination is easily attainable, quick, and often interpreted directly from the workstation. The addition of a contrast-enhanced scan will be at the discretion of the radiologist unless specific contraindication to intravenous administration of contrast exists.

Thunderclap headache refers to a severe and explosive headache with peak intensity within seconds of onset. This has traditionally been recognized as the characteristic feature of subarachnoid hemorrhage from an aneurysm. There have been reports of thunderclap headache in patients with unruptured aneurysm. These are difficult, if not impossible, to detect on non-contrast-enhanced CT.[9]

Non-contrast-enhanced CT is an excellent technique for detecting cerebral or extra-axial hemorrhage, but it can miss an underlying unruptured aneurysm or arteriovenous malformation. These entities can be diagnosed by contrast-enhanced CT or MRI angiography, which are noninvasive alternatives to conventional angiography.

When brain tumor is high on the differential, contrast-enhanced MRI is preferable because of its higher resolution. An additional advantage is that there is no radiation exposure. However, MRI of the brain has a much longer acquisition time, which makes it suboptimal if acute hemorrhage is suspected.

ACUTE CHEST PAIN

Acute onset of chest pain in an otherwise healthy adolescent may be caused by spontaneous pneumothorax or pulmonary embolism. Acute aortic dissection is also in the differential but is extremely rare in the pediatric and adolescent population. Abdominal abnormalities always need to be considered as well.

Primary spontaneous pneumothorax typically occurs in tall thin males aged 10 to 30 years. Cigarette smoking increases the risk. Ninety percent of episodes occur while the patient is at rest. Chest pain and dyspnea are the classic symptoms that often resolve within 24 hours, even if the pneumothorax remains untreated and does not resolve. On physical examination, tachycardia is the most common finding. Decreased breath sounds or increased resonance on percussion are very difficult to detect, because the pneumothorax is often small. Most individuals with spontaneous pneumothorax have unrecognized underlying lung disease, most commonly subpleural blebs.

Chest radiography should be the first investigation performed to assess pneumothorax, because it is simple, inexpensive, rapid, cheap, and noninvasive. A single frontal view with the patient erect is sufficient. An expiratory radiograph may help visualize a small pneumothorax, because the decreased lung volume accentuates the constant volume of air within the pleural space. If the spontaneous pneumothorax is small (involving <15% of the hemithorax) and the patient is minimally symptomatic, high-flow supplemental oxygen will accelerate reabsorption of the air by the pleura. If it is large (>15%–20% of the hemithorax), simple aspiration with a plastic intravenous catheter, thoracentesis catheter, or chest tube is usually successful. Underlying lung disease is best evaluated by non–contrast-enhanced chest CT, which demonstrates ipsilateral bullae or blebs in 89% of patients compared with 20% of control subjects matched for age and smoking status.

Pulmonary embolism is primarily a disease that occurs in patients over the age of 55 years, but it is a recognized entity in the adolescent population and affects girls twice as often as boys. Common complaints include chest pain, dyspnea, cough, and hemoptysis. Common physical findings include hypoxemia and signs of deep vein thrombosis. Major risk factors include estrogen-containing contraceptive use and elective abortion in females and trauma in males. When pulmonary embolism is suspected, a helical CT scan with intravenous contrast should be the initial step in the workup. The embolism appears as a low-density filling defect within the pulmonary artery. Ventilation-perfusion scans in nuclear medicine are used less frequently, because contrast-enhanced CT is more sensitive, is quicker, and does not depend on patient cooperation. Ventilation-perfusion scans are still used on select patients with absolute contraindication to the use of contrast media (documented allergy, severe renal insufficiency, etc).[11]

ACUTE-ONSET SCROTAL PAIN

Acute-onset scrotal pain in the adolescent population could be caused by testicular torsion, which is a potentially devastating condition that cuts off the arterial blood supply to the testis. Delay in diagnosis and treatment can result in testicular necrosis, which necessitates orchidectomy. Diagnostic imaging, particularly Doppler ultrasonography, plays an important role in the assessment of a patient with acute scrotal pain.

Intravaginal testicular torsion occurs most commonly in the peripubertal period, with peak incidence in the 13- to 17-year range. It is associated with a bell-clapper deformity, a congenital anomaly in which the tunica vaginalis completely surrounds the testis, allowing the testicle to twist freely as a result of the absence of normal posterior anchoring.[3] This congenital anomaly occurs in ~12% of males. If testicular torsion is repaired within 6 hours of the initial insult, salvage rates of 80% to 100% are typical. These rates decline to nearly 0% after 24 hours. Approximately 5% to 10% of torsed testes spontaneously detorse, but the risk of retorsion remains high, thus the importance of early diagnosis.[12,13]

The classic presentation of testicular torsion includes acute-onset scrotal pain, scrotal swelling and erythema, and difficulty palpating the testis. History of a previous episode can be recalled in up to 40% of patients. Nausea and vomiting are frequent associated findings.

Differential considerations include acute epididymitis or epididymo-orchitis, abscess, torsion of the epididymal appendix, incarcerated hernia, hematoma, ruptured varicocele, and scrotal tumor.

Preferred examination is ultrasonography with color and power Doppler imaging. Power Doppler is a variant of color Doppler flow imaging in which the strength of the Doppler signal is displayed in color as opposed to the speed and direction of blood flow. It is inherently more sensitive in terms of flow detection than standard color Doppler imaging. Both color Doppler and power Doppler imaging have similar sensitivities for demonstrating flow in small testes, although the combination of both techniques exceeds that of each alone.[12] Overall, the specificity is 77% to 100%, and the sensitivity is 86% to 100%. Normal testes appear relatively symmetric in size with symmetric flow to the testes and epididymis on color or power Doppler. In patients with torsion, testicular enlargement caused by engorgement may be seen. Uniformly hypoechoic testis is seen early on with the later appearance of heterogeneous echotexture, primarily hypoechoic, which usually indicates necrosis. The diagnosis of acute testicular torsion depends on the ability to confirm unequivocally absent blood flow in the painful testis and also to demonstrate normal blood flow in the contralateral asymptomatic testis.[3,12,14]

Findings considered diagnostic of acute epididymo-orchitis include an enlarged hyperemic epididymis and ipsilateral testis. Associated reactive hydrocele and scrotal wall thickening may be present.

MRI is very accurate for identification of testicular torsion, but its use is limited by the length and cost of the examination as well as limited availability in most institutions.

Nuclear scintigraphy was the evaluation of choice before the development of high-resolution ultrasound coupled with color Doppler. This modality is no longer favored, because of the associated radiation and less widespread availability as well as the improved capability of color and power Doppler sonography in the evaluation of perfusion. Nuclear scintigraphy is helpful with indeterminate sonographic findings.[13] Technetium-99m pertechnetate is the agent of choice, and immediate radionuclide angiograms are obtained, which should demonstrate symmetric flow to both testes in the patient without testicular torsion. In prepubescent boys, it is difficult to detect blood flow to the testis by Doppler imaging, so nuclear scintigraphy may be the imaging of choice in this population when testicular torsion is suspected.

LOWER ABDOMINAL OR PELVIC PAIN IN ADOLESCENT GIRLS

Acute-onset lower abdominal or pelvic pain in adolescent girls can be caused by ectopic pregnancy, ovarian torsion, or pelvic inflammatory disease (PID). Ultrasound examination is the imaging study of choice for all 3 of these entities.

Transvaginal sonography allows detailed visualization of the uterus and adnexa, including the ovaries. The fallopian tubes can be visualized only when they are abnormal and distended, usually from postinflammatory obstruction or ectopic pregnancy. Ultrasound is readily available and noninvasive and can be performed at the patient's bedside. In the non–sexually active female, transabdominal pelvic ultrasound is performed by using the urinary bladder as an acoustic window. The ovaries can usually be identified, and the presence of bilateral blood flow can essentially rule out the diagnosis of ovarian torsion.[3]

Laboratory detection of β-human chorionic gonadotropin (β-HCG) is required for the diagnosis of ectopic pregnancy. Although β-HCG levels and their rate of increase may vary with ectopic pregnancies, a negative β-HCG result effectively excludes the diagnosis of intrauterine or extrauterine pregnancy. Clinical presentation varies, but the classic clinical triad includes pain, vaginal bleeding, and an adnexal mass. The clinical triad for ectopic pregnancy is nonspecific and present in <50% of ectopic pregnancies. The positive predictive value of the triad is only 14%.[15]

Risk factors for ectopic pregnancy include previous PID, previous ectopic pregnancy, pregnancy in a woman with an intrauterine device in place, pregnancy achieved by means of in vitro fertilization or fertility drugs, previous tubal surgery (reconstruction or tubal coagulation), cigarette smoking, and increasing age.

In patients with a stable clinical condition, transabdominal and transvaginal sonography can be performed. The demonstration of an intrauterine gestational sac effectively excludes the diagnosis of ectopic pregnancy. A search for a possible ectopic pregnancy as part of a heterotopic pregnancy should be attempted.

With a positive β-HCG level of >1000 IU/mL (2 International Standards standard) or 2000 IU/mL (International Reference Preparation standard), a gestational sac should be identifiable within the uterus on transvaginal sonograms.[3]

If an intrauterine gestational sac is not found, an ectopic pregnancy must be considered. If the patient's β-HCG concentration is below the threshold level and if the only finding is the lack of an intrauterine gestational sac, serial follow-up examinations and β-HCG level determinations are required. A normal intrauterine pregnancy should demonstrate a β-HCG doubling time of 48 hours.

Adnexal torsion requires a quick and confident diagnosis to save the adnexal structures from infarction. The ovary has a dual arterial and venous blood supply. Typically, the ovary and fallopian tube are involved. This condition usually is associated with reduced venous return from the ovary as a result of stromal edema, hyperstimulation, or a mass.

Two groups tend to be affected: women in their mid-20s and women who are postmenopausal. Approximately 20% of the cases of torsion occur during pregnancy. Adolescents, perhaps because of changes in the weight of their maturing adnexa, also are at risk.

Ultrasonography with color Doppler analysis is the method of choice for evaluation of adnexal torsion, because it can show morphologic and physiologic changes in the ovary. Gray-scale and spectral findings are correlated with the age of the torsion (acute versus chronic) and the degree of the twist or torsion.[3,15]

Typically, the affected ovary is enlarged and has multiple immature or small follicles along its periphery. On color Doppler sonograms, no intraovarian venous flow is present; this finding is followed by a lack of intraovarian arterial flow. Flow within the adnexal vessels may be preserved. Rarely, CT or MRI is needed for diagnosis. Contrast-enhanced CT or MRI can serve as a secondary modality when ultrasonographic findings are nondiagnostic.

Ultrasound is the most frequently ordered examination when PID is suspected. The most common ultrasonographic finding for PID is a normal examination. Positive ultrasonographic imaging findings of PID may include a uterus that is ill defined because of inflammation (however, this finding is unusual); central endometrial cavity echo thickening and heterogeneity (endometritis); hydrosalpinx or pyosalpinx; enlarged ovaries with ill-defined margins that often appear adherent to the uterus; and adjacent free fluid that is present in the adnexa or cul-de-sac.[3]

SUSPECTED RENAL STONE

Unenhanced helical CT (UHCT) is a safe, rapidly performed test for the evaluation of suspected renal colic in adolescents. It is highly sensitive and specific for renal and ureteral calculi and, more importantly, allows visualization of alternate pathology.[16] UHCT allows for rapid triage and localization of stones and in most institutions is recommended as the primary diagnostic modality for the evaluation of adolescents with suspected renal colic.[16,17]

On ultrasonography, stones are demonstrated as bright echogenic foci with posterior acoustic shadowing. Stones in the kidneys and the distal ureter at or near the ureterovesicular junction (UVJ) are visualized fairly well with ultrasonography, especially if dilatation is present. In addition, ultrasonography is good for the visualization of complications such as hydronephrosis. However, some patients with acute obstruction have little or no dilation. Absence of the ureteral jet, as visualized with color Doppler on the symptomatic side, is presumptive evidence for a high-grade obstruction in a well-hydrated patient.[3]

Ultrasonography is very insensitive (as low as 24%), especially with stones smaller than 2 mm, stones at the ureteropelvic junction, or stones in the midureter. Compared with UHCT, ultrasonography is operator dependent and more time consuming. Ultrasonography is fairly specific when stones are seen, with a specificity as high as 90%.

With a sensitivity of 94% to 97% and a specificity of 96% to 100%, helical CT is the most sensitive radiologic examination for the detection, localization, and characterization of urinary calcifications. Helical CT scans frequently depict nonobstructing stones that are missed on intravenous pyelography (IVP). CT is faster, and no contrast agent is needed for most patients. CT easily differentiates between nonopaque stones and blood clots or tumors (compared with IVP, which may depict only a filling defect). In addition, helical CT is better than ultrasonography or IVP for detecting other causes of abdominal pain. Therefore, ultrasonography is often skipped in favor of UHCT.

Because stones in the collecting system may be obscured by contrast material, unenhanced CT is usually performed. Because disease may recur, minimizing the radiation dose is critical. The use of intravenous contrast increases the radiation dose of a CT examination. Reported radiation doses for CT are 2.8 to 4.5 mSv compared with 1.3 to 1.5 mSv for a 3-image IVP. However, the uterine dose is ~0.006 Gy for 4-image IVP compared with 0.0046 Gy for unenhanced CT.

One of the pitfalls with non–contrast-enhanced CT is differentiating phleboliths from calculi in the urinary tract. Soft tissue around the rim of a calculus can differentiate it from a phlebolith. A phlebolith may have a comet tail of soft tissue extending from it; this finding helps differentiate it from a calculus. On CT scans, phleboliths do not have radiolucent centers, as often seen on plain radiographs. Phleboliths, which can simulate a stone, are rarely seen during adolescence.

Stones at the UVJ may be difficult to distinguish from stones that have already passed into the bladder. If the distinction changes therapy, a repeat scan through the UVJ in the prone position may be helpful. Stones that have already passed into the bladder will drop into a dependent location.[18]

In an adolescent with suspected stones in the urinary tract, non–contrast-enhanced CT may depict stones in the ureter; enlarged kidneys; hydronephrosis (83% sensitive, 94% specific); perinephric fluid (82% sensitive, 93% specific); ureteral dilatation (90% sensitive, 93% specific); and a soft-tissue rim sign (good positive predictive value).[2]

REFERENCES

1. Doria AS, Moineddin R, Kellenberger CJ, et al. US or CT for diagnosis of appendicitis in children and adults? A meta-analysis. *Radiology.* 2006;241(1):83–94
2. Siegel MJ. *Pediatric Body CT.* Philadelphia, PA: Lippincott, Williams & Wilkens; 1999
3. Siegel MJ. *Pediatric Sonography.* Philadelphia, PA: Lippincott, Williams & Wilkens; 2002
4. Birnbaum BA, Wilson SR. Appendicitis at the millennium. *Radiology.* 2000;215(2):337–348
5. Kaiser S, Frenckner B, Jorulf HK. Suspected appendicitis in children: US and CT—a prospective randomized study. *Radiology.* 2002;223(3):633–638
6. Taylor GA. Suspected appendicitis in children: in search of the single best diagnostic test. *Radiology.* 2004;231(2):293–295
7. Lewis DW. Headaches in children and adolescents. *Am Fam Physician.* 2002;65(4):625–632
8. Miller J. Headache: when is neuroimaging needed? *Radiol Rounds.* 2003;1(4):1–3
9. Dodick DW. Thunderclap headache. *J Neurol Neurosurg Psychiatry.* 2002;72(1):6–11
10. Lewis DW, Qureshi F. Acute headache in children and adolescents presenting to the emergency department. *Headache.* 2000;40(3):200–203
11. Bozlar U, Gaughen JR, Nambiar AP, Hagspiel KD. Imaging diagnosis of acute pulmonary embolism. *Expert Rev Cardiovasc Ther.* 2007;5(3):519–529
12. Gunther P, Schenk JP, Wunsch R, et al. Acute testicular torsion in children: the role of sonography in the diagnostic workup. *Eur Radiol.* 2006;16(11):2527–2532
13. Ringdahl E, Teague L. Testicular torsion. *Am Fam Physician.* 2006;74(10):1739–1743
14. Aso C, Enríquez G, Fité M, et al. Gray-scale and color Doppler sonography of scrotal disorders in children: an update. *Radiographics.* 2005;25(5):1197–1214
15. Patel MD. "Rule out ectopic": asking the right questions, getting the right answers. *Ultrasound Q.* 2006;22(2):87–100
16. Colistro R, Torreggiani WC, Lyburn ID, et al. Unenhanced helical CT in the investigation of acute flank pain. *Clin Radiol.* 2002;57(6):435–441
17. Smith RC, Varanelli M. Diagnosis and management of acute ureterolithiasis: CT is truth. *AJR Am J Roentgenol.* 2000;175(1):3–6
18. Lumerman J, Gershbaum MD, Hines J, Nardi P, Beuchert P, Katz DS. Unenhanced helical computed tomography for the evaluation of suspected renal colic in the adolescent population: a pilot study. *Urology.* 2001;57(2):342–346

A

Abstinence, sexual, 70, 73, 74–76, 81

Active listening, as communication skill, 8

Adherence
communicating with adolescents about, 4–5
definition of, 99–100
demographic and socioeconomic factors, 104–107
interventions, 107–110
measures of, 101–103
scope of the problem, 101
in specific diseases, 110–114

Adherence in adolescents: a review of the literature, **99–118**

Adnexal torsion, 197

Adverse effects, as factor in medication adherence, 104, 107

AECG monitoring, 177–179

Affirmations, in motivational interviewing, 57, 70, 71

Agenda setting, in motivational interviewing, 58, 60, 73

Airway reactivity, assessing, 157–161

Alcohol use
helping to stop, role of primary care clinician, 88–91
reduction, effectiveness of motivational interviewing, 62–63, 69

Amenorrhea, 18, 20, 25, 36

Anorexia nervosa, 18, 34, 169

Antipsychotics, 176

Antiretroviral agents, 100, 110–111

Antitreponemal antibody testing, 141–142

Anxiety, 37, 44

Appendicitis, suspected, 190–192

Arrhythmias, 177, 178–179, 180, 184, 187

Arterial blood gas, 163–164

Assertiveness, 10

Asthma
medication adherence, 100, 107, 110, 112
pulmonary function testing, 147–149, 158–159, 161

Athletic populations, screening tests, 176–177

Autonomy, 2–5, 55, 56, 81

B

Behavioral concerns, talking with adolescents and their families about, 41–53

Behavioral strategies, for medication adherence, 108–109

Behavior-change plans, use of, in motivational interviewing, 58, 60, 62

Binge eating, 4, 18, 31–34

Body image, 34–36

Body language, making use of, 12–13

Borrelia burgdorfei, 143

Bronchial challenge testing, 158–161

Bronchodilator testing, 157–158

Bulimia nervosa, 4, 6, 19, 34

C

Cancer, teens living with
communicating with, 119–134
pulmonary function testing, 156
treatment adherence, 110

Carbon monoxide diffusing capacity, 155–157

Cardiac catheterization, 166, 186–187

Cardiac testing in adolescents, **169–192**

Cardiopulmonary exercise testing, 162

Cardiovascular disease
cardiac stress test, 162

cardiovascular MRI, 187
echocardiography, 187
Holter monitoring, 180

Chemotherapy, 121, 159

Chest pain
acute, imaging studies, 196–197
evaluation of, 170–174, 177, 180, 182
pulmonary function testing, 149, 150, 159, 163

Chest radiography, 188–189, 197

Cigarette smoking, 15–16, 64, 69, 197, 199

Cocaine use, 96, 174

Cognitive status, 5–6

Collaboration, as feature of motivational interviewing, 55–56

Communicating with teens who are living with cancer, **119–134**

Communication skills, during medical interviews, 7–8

Compliance. see *Adherence*

Computed tomography (CT)
adnexal torsion, 197
cardiac testing, 169, 188–189
headache, 193
lung disease, 197
suspected appendicitis, 193
suspected renal stone, 202

Condom use, 69, 73, 76, 79

Confidentiality
discussion of mental health problems, 43–46
importance of, in conducting medical interviews, 4, 10
interviewing adolescents with eating disorders, 21–22
questions regarding substance use, 96–97

Consistency, as communication skill, 8

Contraception, hormonal, medication adherence, 104, 112–113

Contraceptive behaviors, motivational interviewing and, 69–82

Control issues, 3

Cough, 149, 150, 160

Counseling techniques, for medication adherence, 110

CRAFFT (screening tool), 83–84, 88, 90–97

Cystic fibrosis, 151, 152, 157, 159, 167

Cytomegalovirus, 135, 147

D

Daily journals, 8, 10

Decisional balance, in motivational interviewing, 58–59

Decision-making
capacity, of adolescents, 46
shared, teens living with cancer, 127–129

Demographic factors, impact on adherence, 104–107

Depression, 37, 106

Dextromethorphan, 95

Diabetes
care, effectiveness of motivational interviewing, 62, 64
treatment adherence, 100, 104, 106, 110, 113–114

Dietary history, in eating-disorder assessments, 25–27

Directly observed therapy, 110

Discrepancy, developing, 56

Doppler ultrasonography, 193, 194, 197

Drug and metabolite levels, monitoring, as measure of adherence, 101

Drug use
helping to stop, role of primary care clinician, 83–98
prevention, effectiveness of motivational interviewing, 62, 63–64

Dyspnea, 150, 159, 161, 165, 167, 197

E

Eating disorder, not otherwise specified, DSM-IV criteria, 19, 34

Eating-disorder behaviors, 27–34, 62, 64

Eating disorders
anorexia nervosa, 18, 34, 172
bradycardia in, 172
bulimia nervosa, 4, 6, 19, 34
interviewing adolescents with, 18–40

Echocardiography, 170, 182–184

Ectopic pregnancy, 196–197

Educational strategies, for medication adherence, 109

Egocentrism, 5–6

Electrocardiography, 169–191
 evaluation of chest pain, 173–177
 evaluation of QT interval, 178–179
 interpretation of abnormal heart rate and rhythm, 170–173
 monitoring, stress testing with, 183
 use in sports participants' screening, 179–180

Electronic drug monitoring, as measure of adherence, 101

Electrophysiology study, 186–187

Elicit-provide-elicit, in motivational interviewing, 58, 79–81

Emergency contraception, 70, 79

Emotional concerns, talking with adolescents and their families about, 41–53

Empathy, expressing, 56, 79

Empowerment, teens living with cancer, 127–129

End of life, teens living with cancer, 131–132

Epstein-Barr virus, 135, 136–137

Exercise
 adolescents with eating disorders, 29–31
 exercise-induced bronchoconstriction, 165

Exercise testing, 165–166, 179–183

F

Family history, eating-disorder assessments, 37

Flexibility, as communication skill, 8

Food restriction, 29

Food rituals, 29

FRAMES paragraph, 58, 60, 61, 78–79

G

GAPS form, 13, 14

H

Headaches, imaging studies, 192–193

HEADS (screening tool), 14

Heart disease, cardiac testing, 166–189

Heart rate, abnormal, interpretation of, 167–170

Heart rhythm, abnormal, interpretation of, 167–170

Helical CT, 192, 194, 198

Helping adolescents to stop using drugs: role of the primary care clinician, **83–98**

Hemoptysis, 197

Hepatitis A, 136, 139

Hepatitis B, 139–140, 142

Hepatitis C, 135, 141

Hepatitis D, 142

Hepatitis E, 142

Hepatitis testing, 139

Heterophile antibody test, 136–138

Holter monitoring, 173, 180–181

Homicidality, 37, 46

Hopelessness, solution-focused interventions, 49–51

Human immunodeficiency virus (HIV)
 as cause of infectious mononucleosis, 136, 138
 CMV morbidity and mortality, 138
 medication adherence, 100, 104, 105, 107, 110–112
 serological diagnosis, 136–138
 syphilis coinfection, 143

Hydronephrosis, 201–202

Hypertension, 100, 104–105

Hypoxia, 166–172

I

Identity, 5

Imaginary audience, 6

Imaging in adolescent medicine, **193–202**

Importance and confidence rulers, in motivational interviewing, 58, 59–60, 76–78

Infectious diseases, serological diagnosis of, 135–148

Infectious mononucleosis, 136–138

Information giving, teens living with cancer, 121–125

Internet, as source of health care information, 122, 125

Interviewing the adolescent with an eating disorder, **18–40**

Intravenous contrast material, 195

Intravenous pyelography, 201

Introduction to interviewing: the art of communicating with adolescents, **1–17**

K

Kidneys, enlarged, 201–202

Kidney stones, 202

L

Lower abdominal pain, in adolescent girls, 194, 199–201

Lung disease, 149, 197

Lung volumes, 151–158

Lyme disease, 146

M

Magnetic resonance imaging (MRI)
  adnexal torsion, 200
  angiography, 196
  cardiac testing, 169, 188–189
  testicular torsion, 198

Marijuana use, 63–64, 85, 92–93

Mature minor, concept of, 128

Medical history, eating-disorder assessments, 36

Medical interviews
  communication skills, 7–8
  techniques for enhancing information-sharing, 8–13
  tools for structuring, 13–16

Medication use, by adolescents with eating disorders, 34

Menstrual history, eating-disorder assessments, 16, 36

Mental health
  adolescents' knowledge of, 41–43
  referral, as adherence intervention, 109–110

Mental illness, impact on medication adherence, 104, 106, 109–110

Methacholine challenge testing, 161–164

Mnemonics, 13–16, 83

Mononucleosis, infectious, 136–138

Monospot test, 136, 137

Motivational interviewing
  with adolescents, 54–68
  helping adolescents to stop using drugs, 87–88
  sexual and contraceptive behaviors and, 69–82

Motivational interviewing and sexual and contraceptive behaviors, **69–82**

Motivational interviewing with adolescents, **54–68**

Myelodysplasia, 123, 127

Myocardial infarction, 170, 174, 178

Myocardial ischemia, 176

N

Neurally mediated hypotension (NMH), 184–186

Neuroimaging studies, for headache, 196

Nonjudgmental approach, as communication skill, 7

Nuclear scintigraphy, 199

O

Obsessive-compulsive disorder, 29

Open-ended questions, in motivational interviewing, 57, 70–71

Orchidectomy, 197

Organ transplant recipients
  CMV morbidity and mortality, 136
  medication adherence, 104, 107, 110, 112
  testing for HCV infection, 142

Ovarian cyst, 194

Ovarian torsion, 194, 199

Over-the-counter medications, misuse of, 85, 93–95

PACES (screening tool), 14–16
Palpitations, 170–181
Passive-aggressive behavior, 10
Patient-provider relationship, as factor in medication adherence, 108
Peak expiratory flow rate, 149
Pediatricians, role in cancer care, 119, 121–122
Pelvic inflammatory disease (PID), 199–200
Pelvic pain, in adolescent girls, 193–199
Pericarditis, 171–173
Permission, asking, in motivational interviewing, 58, 80
Personal fable, 6
Pharmacy refills, checking, as measure of adherence, 102
Phleboliths, 201–202
Physical examinations, routine, 2
Pill counts, as measure of adherence, 101
Pneumothorax, spontaneous, 196, 197
Positron-emitting tracers (PET), 189–190
Pregnancy
adnexal torsion during, 200
ectopic pregnancy, 199–200
motivational interviewing, 69, 78–79
Prescription medications, misuse of, 85, 93–95
Primary care clinicians, role of, helping adolescents to stop using drugs, 83–98
Primary care physicians, role of, communicating with teens living with cancer, 119–126
Psychiatric history and treatments, eating-disorder assessments, 36–37
Psychosocial factors, impact on adherence, 106–107
Pubertal status, 1–2
Pulmonary embolism, 197
Pulmonary function testing in the adolescent, **149–168**

Pulse oximetry, 165–166
Purging behaviors. see *Vomiting, self-induced*

Q

QT interval, evaluation of, 172–179, 191

R

Radiation therapy, 156
Radiography. see *Chest radiography*
Rapid plasma regain (RPR) screening test, 141, 142
Rapport
building, with teens living with cancer, 125–127
strategies for establishing, 57–58, 70–73, 125–127
Reference values, in pulmonary function testing, 153–154
Reflections, in motivational interviewing, 57, 70, 71, 72
Reflective responses, use of, as interview technique, 10
Renal stone, suspected, 201
Resistance, rolling with, 56–57, 65

S

Screening questionnaires, 8, 13
Scrotal pain, acute-onset, 197–198
Self-awareness, as communication skill, 7
Self-efficacy, supporting, 56, 57, 79
Self-harm behaviors, 4, 37
Self-induced vomiting, 34
Self-report, as measure of adherence, 102–103
Serological diagnosis of infectious diseases in the adolescent, **135–148**
Sexual behaviors, motivational interviewing and, 62, 64, 69–82
Sexually transmitted diseases
hepatitis C, 135, 141–142
HIV infection, 135, 144–145
motivational interviewing, 69, 76–78
syphilis, 106, 141–142

Sickle cell disease, 151, 157, 158
Sleep apnea, 167
Smoking. see *Cigarette smoking*
Socioeconomic factors, impact on adherence, 104–107
Solution-focused interventions, 49–51
Spirometry, 149–153
Sports participants, screening tests, 180
Stress testing, 183
Substance use
  adolescents with eating disorders, 34
  communicating with adolescents about, 16
  as factor in medication adherence, 106, 109–110
  helping to stop, role of primary care clinician, 83–98
  motivational interviewing and, 62–64, 69
Suicidality, 37, 46
Summaries and summarizing statements, 11–12, 57, 58, 70, 71
Syncope, 169–170, 177, 180, 181–182
Syphilis, 107, 141–142

T

Talking with adolescents and their families about emotional and behavioral concerns, **41–53**
Testicular torsion, 197–199

Thunderclap headache, 196
Tilt-table testing, 181–182
Tobacco use. see *Cigarette smoking*
Transabdominal sonography, 194
Transvaginal sonography, 199, 200

U

Ultrasonography
  acute-onset scrotal pain, 198, 199
  adnexal torsion, 200
  suspected appendicitis, 193
  suspected renal stone, 201
Unenhanced helical CT (UHCT), 200
Urinary calcifications, 200–201

V

Venereal Disease Research Laboratory test, 141
Ventilation-perfusion scans, 197
Viral hepatitis, 138–143
Vomiting, self-induced, 34

W

Weight-control measures, adolescents with eating disorders, 27
Weight history, eating-disorder assessments, 25
Western blot assay, 145
Wheezing, 149, 160–167